"This is a great handbook!
So much useful information presented in such an
organized and easy-to-use format."

—Martha Clayton Cottrell, M.D.
Physician and author

"Shiatsu has such an incredible effect
on the body . . . it's almost as fun
to give as it is to receive."

—Mary Steenburgen
Academy Award-winning actress

"This lean volume has helped me
cut all the fat out of my teaching."

—Edward Spencer
Acupressure Institute, Berkeley

"The future of health care is in your hands.
This book covers all the important
preventative measures for health and healing."

—Michael Ingraham, M.D., Ph.D., B.Sc.
Natural Health Center, Nassau, Bahamas

THE SHIATSU HANDBOOK

A GUIDE TO THE TRADITIONAL ART OF SHIATSU ACUPRESSURE

SHIZUKO YAMAMOTO
PATRICK McCARTY

Avery Publishing Group

Garden City Park, New York

The medical and health procedures in this book are based on the training, personal experiences, and research of the author. Because each person and situation is unique, the editor and the publisher urge the reader to check with a qualified health professional before using any procedure where there is any question as to its appropriateness.

The publisher does not advocate the use of any particular diet or exercise program but believes the information presented in this book should be available to the public.

Because there is always some risk involved, the author and publisher are not responsible for any adverse effects or consequences resulting from the use of any of the suggestions, preparations, or procedures in this book. Please do not use the book if you are unwilling to assume the risk. Feel free to consult a physician or other qualified health professional. It is a sign of wisdom, not cowardice, to seek a second or third opinion.

Cover Design: William Gonzalez
Interior Illustrations: Susan Reid
Interior Photographs: Mark Oliver
Printer: Paragon Press, Honesdale, PA

Cataloging-in-Publication Data

Yamamoto, Shizuko, 1924–
    The shiatsu handbook : a guide to the traditional art of
    acupressure / Shizuko Yamamoto & Patrick McCarty. — Garden City
    Park, NY : Avery Pub. Group, 1996.
        p.   cm.
    Includes index.
    Rev. ed. of: Macrobiotic family health care and shiatsu, 1985.
    ISBN 0-89529-714-0

    1. Acupressure.   2. Macrobiotic diet.   3. Family—Health and
    hygiene.   4. Holistic medicine.   I. McCarty, Patrick, 1947–   II.
    Title.

RM723.A27Y35   1996   615.8'22
                                             QBI95-2356

Printed in the United States of America

10   9   8   7   6   5   4   3   2   1

Contents

DEDICATION

To our Parents, Sisters and Brothers, Mr. and Mrs. Ohsawa, and
all mankind, without whom we could not have learned
the things we know.

Significance of Illustrations at Chapter Beginnings

PINE-BAMBOO-PLUM (*SHO-CHIKU-BAI*)

In traditional Japanese culture, some common plants have represented many of the traits that are valued by people. The pine, bamboo and plum are examples of such plants that are not only beautiful but also bring to mind positive human qualities.

The Chinese pronounciation for pine, bamboo and plum is *Sho, Chiku* and *Bai* respectively. In Japanese they are called *matsu, take* and *ume* but when the three are together only the Chinese name of *Sho-Chiku-Bai* is used. Currently these symbols are found on many traditional Japanese crafts such as ceramic pottery, sushi dishware, kimono clothing and doorway curtains. *Sho-Chiku-Bai,* arouses a feeling of tradition. It promotes an immense sense of being linked with nature. It reminds one of highly prized and admirable qualities. *Sho-Chiku-Bai* symbolizes deep, inner strength.

PINE *(SHO)*

The pine tree with its evergreen needles symbolizes stability and strength. The tree's ability to spring back to its original position, even after strong winds have affected it, display its durability and strength.

BAMBOO *(CHIKU)*

The bamboo plant symbolizes flexibility and straightness. After the ravages of a typhoon the bamboo remains standing, its flexibilty protecting it. No matter how bamboo is cut it always remains straight.

PLUM *(BAI)*

At the first break of early spring, even when snow is present, the plum will blossom. The plum tree is very hearty and is the first to bloom. Plums have an ancient curative use. For these reasons the plum symbolizes strength.

Preface

There are many books available which explain the techniques on how to give massage. Technique is important, yet, it seems to me, it is essential to understand the foundations which create health and illness in order to successfully apply treatment. Why do we become sick and unhappy? Without a positive change in our understanding, we are destined to repeat past mistakes—we are destined to be ill. Technique alone will not make a significant difference in our overall physical and mental health.

Over seventeen years ago my interest in natural healing led me to the study of shiatsu and macrobiotics. While attending a week long program sponsored by the Kushi Foundation of Brookline, MA, I discovered an interesting type of oriental massage called shiatsu. It was in this class my study of natural healing began. The teacher, a woman with tremendous energy and a charismatic personality, repeatedly emphasized the importance of living in accordance with nature. She stressed that the techniques that we were learning in class must harmonize with the greater forces outside ourselves. Because of her clarity and conviction I was convinced but I really didn't know what she meant by "live with nature." It was only later, after some years and several series of classes, that the subtle wisdom of her simple explanation began to make sense. That teacher was Shizuko Yamamoto—macrobiotic counsellor, exquisite chef, and shiatsu teacher and practitioner.

I was fortunate to work with Ms. Yamamoto on her first book, *Barefoot Shiatsu*. It was written as a textbook to introduce shiatsu to the public. A landmark in its field, it consists of technique and therapy to promote effective treatment. Included are many corrective exercises, a large section on diagnosis, and specific suggestions for both giver and receiver.

Since that book was completed Ms. Yamamoto's technique has evolved. It has become simpler. Instead of adding, she has been substracting—maximizing effect, while minimizing effort. Over the years she has developed a unique macrobiotic consultation. From her extensive experience in the healing field, her consultation has developed into a blend of dietary information, shiatsu treatment, and intuitive understanding of the cause of an individual's problem. Basing her advice and treatment on objective observations, she encourages individuals to understand the cause of their illness or unhappiness and points out natural means to fulfill the goal of making a change for the better.

The idea for this book was first discussed at a beach party in Massachusetts outside of Boston, during a North American Macrobiotic Congress. Because of the success of *Barefoot Shiatsu*, Ms. Yamamoto and I felt that our work was done. That is, we felt that a comprehensive holistic approach to shiatsu was now available to whomever wanted it. However, dozens of shiatsu practitioners felt otherwise. Once they were exposed to the simplicity of *Barefoot Shiatsu* they wanted more. We decide, after much thought, that another shiatsu book which included more about natural healing was needed to satisfy the many enthusiatists who were asking for one. We began work in the Netherlands—at the European Macrobiotic Assembly in Amsterdam. However, as our ideas started to develop, it was evident that our simple vision for the book had expanded into a somewhat larger view. Months passed and we met at several locations where our schedules put us both at the same time. In Holland, New York, Switzerland, Spain, and Eureka, California we taught classes, treated people, and recorded the results. Eventually, our goal of completing such a book was accomplished. Our aim was to create a concise book on natural healing based on actual experience that reduces confusion and suffering and promotes a preventive attitude toward health. We hope we have succeeded in this aim.

This book is not a huge encyclopedia of extensive natural healing practices—but it is a practical guide that can be useful to the whole family. From the beginning chapters on the history of shiatsu and an introduction to macrobiotics, yin/yang theory, and the fundamentals of health, through the application of diet, shiatsu, breathing and other time-tested remedies, you will find thoretical and practical information at your fingertips. It is our hope that this book will help you to strengthen the world family physically and spiritually and will be useful for many years to come.

Our appreciation is extended to the following people who were most helpful in making this book possible. Special thanks go to Susan Reid for the detailed illustrations which add so much to the beauty of the book. Mark Oliver created photographs which display not only clarity but activity and spirit. Joanne Sullivan shared valuable comments and preliminary editing skills, Susan Stearns devoted herself in the final editing which added clarity and conciseness to our ideas, Yukiko Iino translated chapters which were originally written in Japanese, Cynthia Ann Noble created the artwork at the beginning of each section, and to my wife, Meredith, who gave nourishment, both physical and emotional, during the many months of labor. We also owe a debt of gratitude to those students and patients whose questions and needs stimulated the writing of *The SHIATSU Handbook.*

Patrick McCarty

Introduction

This is a practical book that will help you gain and maintain vibrant health. It will assist you in providing natural, time tested healing techniques for yourself and your family. It is a holistic guide which bases the foundation of health on nature and the unity of body, mind, and spirit. We are responsible for our own health. Unifying the aspects of individuality, body, mind, and spirit stabilizes and strengthens each one of us. This book gives you the tools and understanding to maintain or regain your natural birthright. Your family's and your own health is in your hands.

Healing practices have developed as a response to human suffering. As time passes, health and medical care have become increasingly complicated. Reliance on specialists has become the standard approach. Where once there was the general family doctor, now we have specialists such as the cardiologist (heart), urologist (bladder and kidney), ophthalmologist (eye), otolaryngologist (ear, nose, and throat), dermatologist (skin), gastroenterologist (digestive system), pulmonary specialist (lungs), orthopedist (bone and joint), gynecologist (women's problems), neurologist (nerve), endocrinologist (hormones/metabolic function), oncologist (cancer) and psychiatrist (mental and emotional problems). Each is concerned with disease and illness of one part of your body. Many people go from specialist to specialist in search of a name for their illness and relief from their symptoms. This process is a recent one. It began only a little more than one hundred years ago. Nowadays, the underlying theory which guides the choice and type of treatment has turned away from its ancient beginnings. Instead of making humankind whole, it deals with diseased parts.

In the distant past, Hippocrates and others, felt that humans were part of nature. The goal of medicine was prevention. It was thought that as people violated natural law, they became sick. The aim of treatment was to allow the patient to re-establish the previous state of balance. Therefore the medical person, the patient, and the treatment followed the way of nature.

It is easy to be impressed with newly developed technologies, but we sometimes forget about the underlying reasons for such development. Which is of more interest to us, the high degree of sophistication in dentistry—with the noiseless drills, anesthetics, and artificial tooth replacements—or the rotten state of our teeth?

Present day medicine relies heavily on technology for both the diagnosis and treatment of the patient. Although necessary at times, this approach is expensive and takes the responsibility of healing away from the individual. Because of the complicated nature of modern medicine, many people feel that their personal health care is out of their hands.

This handbook gives you the confidence to know when and how you can treat yourself. It also tells you when it may be necessary to call in the help of a specialist. Putting choice in health care back into your hands is one of our aims.

The highest goal of living is to become a good person. A good person is one that is happy and contributes to others. If this is your honest aim, then you will automatically become a good husband, wife or child. Thinking how someone else feels before you act helps contribute to healthy relationships. If you desire to help and serve others, then you will have a useful life. In this life no special techniques are necessary. All that is necessary is your sincere wish to be happy and useful.

In this society, we have lost this aim to help others. Instead, our motivation to act comes from the desire for money, personal recognition or private pleasure. Current education trains children to become technicians, emphasis is placed on learning techniques. However, in reality, techniques don't matter much. Do you need a technique to love your children? Is a technique necessary to enjoy the sunset or a good book? We should train to develop ourselves as sensitive people, open and aware of life around us. Our lives are enriched as we learn to understand the way of nature.

The Shiatsu Handbook is divided into three sections. The first section of this handbook, *Foundation*, lays the groundwork so we can understand the way that nature operates. The History of Shiatsu along with Macrobiotics, the large view of life, are introduced, and the macrobiotic way of applying natural methods in our everyday activities is explained. The underlying principles of the cause of illness and the natural forces that affect all of us are also explained. Furthermore, the fundamental areas that create our health and happiness are discussed in detail. From observing natural events, the working of the healing process becomes clear. The treatment that we use never cures the patient. It is the patient who cures him or herself.

Section two, *Tools*, gives you the practical means, such as shiatsu (finger pressure), to accomplish the goal of alleviating suffering and becoming a more sensitive person. Shiatsu and the other tools that we use are based on longtime tradition and our current experience in treating thousands of people. They complement the healing process. Here, two main areas will be discussed in detail: advice before the treatment; and how to give a complete shiatsu-acupressure session.

The third section of the handbook, *Balance*, shows specific treatments for some of the most common family complaints. Fatigue, headaches, arthritis, asthma, common cold, high blood pressure, allergies, sciatica, hay fever, and many more health problems are discussed in depth. Emotional problems and first aid are included as well.

You may be doing many of the suggestions in this book already. However, even if your are making just a little mistake in any area of life, you may continue to have trouble. Each person must discover what is proper for oneself in diet, exercise and outlook on life. With this discovery, your personal training will develop by itself.

An adventure that should continue throughout life is the study of nature and all of its wonders. If we take natural phenomena for granted, we miss the pleasure of many of the interesting things life has to offer. Neglecting the study of nature leaves us without a deep understanding of how life works. This neglect has helped to create our illness.

The purpose of *The Shiatsu Handbook* is to awaken our understanding of nature. It is our hope that the macrobiotic principle of balance, when applied to shiatsu, diet and exercise, will come alive for you. With the obvious physical changes that occur with this form of natural healing, we can learn not only practical solutions to body troubles but we can also gain insight into the process of life. The personal experience of symptom relief is important in order to demonstrate the power of self-healing. Simultaneously, the treatments in this handbook will promote understanding of life's experiences within each individual as well as within the family. The application of this easy-to-do system is designed to be used by all people.

Husbands can treat wives, parents can treat children, children can treat grandparents, and friends can treat friends. In this way, healthy bodies are made and family unity is encouraged. In a very practical sense, we can renew our physical and mental health and restore our independence. And it can be accomplished easily, simply, and, most of all, naturally.

Foundation
Pine

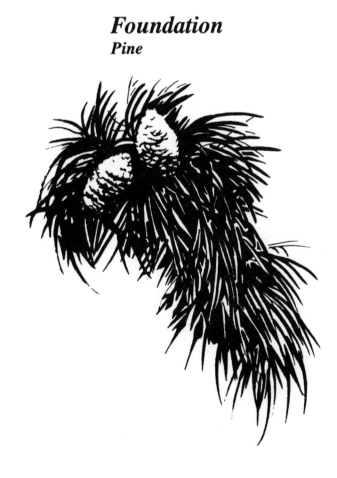

History of Shiatsu

Today, shiatsu, acupuncture and moxibustion are becoming more prevalent all over the world. Scientists and medical practitioners from both East and West are conducting research and publishing books on shiatsu, while an increasing number of people are seeking shiatsu treatment.

The origin of the Japanese word "shiatsu" is not certain. Over the centuries, information that make up the shiatsu techniques was gathered through trial and error. The healing techniques that are fundamental to shiatsu probably originated in ancient China, and later came to Japan. Shiatsu is a synthesis of Judo principles, Do-In (self massage), and ancient massage. It is an evolving process derived from the unique experience of healers. The first syllable in shiatsu, *shi* means fingers and the second, *atsu* indicates pressure. Therefore, shiatsu means "to apply pressure on the body with the fingers." Recently in the West, it has become known as acupressure.

It is only recently that the Japanese government became interested in and recognized shiatsu as a complementary medical practice. In 1955, the Japanese parliament adopted a bill on revised *Amma* treatment (ancient Oriental massage). Thus, for the first time in Japan, shiatsu was given official endorsement. Along with

Amma and massage, which had already received recognition, shiatsu was thereafter legally and officially taught in schools.

To better understand shiatsu, we can compare it with two other healing techniques that involve the touch of a practitioner's hands. These two forms are *Amma* and massage (of Western origin). Let's examine the theory, practical application, and historical background of these techniques.

Amma (ancient Oriental massage) originated in ancient China and later was introduced to Japan. The first syllable in *Amma. Am,* denotes pressure and non-pressure, and the second, *ma,* means rubbing. *Amma* is a technique of pressing and rubbing the body. During the early part of the Nara Period (672-707 A.D.), *Amma* was recognized by the official medical authorities. Sometime later it lost popularity and in the Edo Period (1501-1857), it was revived once again. In 1793, a comprehensive handbook on *Amma* was completed. It was one component of the Oriental healing arts. Its working principles are based on theories of meridians (channels of energy) and pressure points.

As far back as the 4th or 5th century B.C., written records indicate that Hippocrates, the father of modern Western medicine, advocated massage. In the ensuing years, records prove that interest still remained, but in small degree. As the Renaissance flourished in France during the latter half of the 16th century, massage was revived. Only in the late 1880's was it introduced to Japan, during the middle of the Meiji Period. Although the word "massage" is French, it is derived from Arabic, Greek, and/or Hebrew and denotes "rubbing, kneading, touching, etc." In today's medical world, massage is used as a complementary treatment in widely ranging applications for general health maintenance.

Amma, deeply embedded in the Oriental approach, and "massage," of Western origin, took different courses in their conceptual development. Each evolved by modifying its weaknesses and exploring its strengths. However, there is a strong tendency to consider the two methods as having the same type of applications. Since both *Amma* and massage have been fully assimilated into Japanese practice, they are administered together rather than independent of each other. In the hands of highly experienced and intuitive practitioners, distinguishing *Amma* from massage techniques becomes especially difficult.

In the Edo Period, the majority of *Amma* practitioners were blind, and they gave treatments in their patients' homes. By the time Western massage was introduced in the late 1880's, there existed many vocational schools of *Amma* for the blind all over Japan. Both *Amma* and massage were taught mostly to this group. Just as the performance of certain Japanese musical instruments was dominated by blind players and therefore, because of their visual limitation did not develop to a high degree, so the development of *Amma* technique stopped and it became a mere tool for comfort and relaxation.

Unlike *Amma*, shiatsu was further refined in its working principles and applications. In the beginning of the Taisho Period (1920's), shiatsu practitioners adopted some body work principles popular in America (such as chiropractic, occupational therapy, etc.). Mr. Namikoshi and the late Mr. Masunaga are but a few examples of excellent practitioners who continued their research. As a result, today, shiatsu represents Oriental " body work." *Amma* and massage also fall into this category.

In analyzing these three healing techniques, it is clear that all are based on the laws of dynamics. This is a study of motion and reaction produced by external forces. One law states that if an object exerts a force on another, there is an equal and opposite force or reaction on the first object by the second. Likewise, when stimulation is applied to the body either in the form of pressing, rubbing, or kneading, the body accordingly produces some internal changes. Detecting these internal reactions, an experienced practitioner then applies other stimulation, which is based on one's intuitive reactions to the internal changes in one's patient. Thus, a practitioner of these techniques applies dynamic stimulation to the patient. All three massage methods promote the circulation of body fluids and regulate the functions of the organs. Physiological reactions to this dynamic stimulation follow the same basic route. In the case of shiatsu, the application of energy-force is at one point applied, for example, with the thumb. The pressure is administered rhythmically in varying degrees, so that the recipient feels the compound results of varying applications of pressure. The direct administration of pressure in shiatsu is simpler and more linear than in the other two techniques.

Neither a thorough physical check-up by a doctor of Western medicine, nor a complete laboratory analysis, can adequately diagnose and cure symptoms caused by nervous and mental disorders and the imbalance of the autonomic nervous system. Shiatsu, together with other forms of massage, is a system which has developed from centuries of experience, and has proven effective in curing many symptoms. Among these symptoms are headaches, dizziness, ringing in the ears, eye-strain, general fatigue, stiff neck and shoulders, lower backache, constipation, numbness of limbs, chills, flushes, insomnia, and lack of appetite. Shiatsu and related techniques have also proven effective for curing chronic and painful conditions such as high blood pressure, rheumatism, and general neuralgia.

Shiatsu practitioners have long been considered authorities on treating minor diseases in Japan. In general, the Japanese public favors shiatsu treatment and, for many years, these practitioners have played a major role in health maintenance. The previously mentioned forms of massage and shiatsu are wonderful tools for the betterment of health. With the fact that life is forever changing, even these techniques must continue to evolve.

The practice of eating large amounts of animal food has created bodies that are very tight and rigid. In order to effectively deal with this hard, stiff situation an appropriate shiatsu technique naturally evolved. The "Macrobiotic or Barefoot Shiatsu" style developed as a response to the western condition. It is a technique that deals with the common problems that numerous westerners have. When someone is tight, they need a vigorous style of treatment to loosen them up. Anything less than this will be ineffective and often a waste of time. Don't forget, however, that the aim of treatment is to create balance within the individual. We are always attentive to the needs of the receiver.

This style of shiatsu coordinates the breathing of the giver and the receiver as an important part of the treatment. Breathing together creates a lot of energy which is used in the correcting process. A vigorous style, which includes not only pressing with the thumbs but the use of the giver's whole body, helps to loosen up the stiffness that so many people have. Stretching is also an important part of this style. In the diagnosis segment of a shiatsu treatment the senses of touch, vision and smell are used. (see *Barefoot Shiatsu*, by the same author for more complete details on diagnosis). By understanding the imbalances that are present, accurate way of life recommendations can be made. Recommendations that include diet, breathing and movement exercises, and way of thinking are combined with the shiatsu treatment. In this way the individual can be guided toward wholeness. These methods are used because they are effective. After so many years of treating people we have realized that this style of shiatsu, which deals with the aspects of everyday living, promotes the fastest recovery from illness and suffering. It is also good for the one who gives the treatment.

Macrobiotics

At first glance, Macrobiotics appears to be a new wholistic health system. However, the word macrobiotics was used many centuries ago to describe people who were healthy and lived a long time. "Macro" means "great" or "large" and "bios" means "life." Macrobiotics is the art of living a long and happy life according to the principles of nature. The essence of macrobiotics has existed for thousands of years. More recently, around the turn of the century, these natural principles were revitalized and reintroduced by George Ohsawa. Mr. Ohsawa taught the principles of the Order of the Universe extensively in Japan, India, Africa, Europe, and the United States. His wife Mrs. Lima Ohsawa continues to teach in Tokyo. Many of his students including Shizuko Yamamoto present this ancient information to modern people. Borrowing its ancient name, this traditional information is again called Macrobiotics.

The macrobiotic approach to shiatsu is based on the timeless principles of change. This approach is a unique blend of Eastern and Western natural health and medical influences. It uses healing methods that are simple, rational, and effective, yet have no ill effects on the user.

The body has its own healing process which involves the blood, nerves, tissues, and immune function. Only remedies that assist our body and direct nature in her efforts to allow us to heal ourselves and strenghten our defense mechanism can be called natural or true remedies.

The use of diet, including proper cooking, plus shiatsu, exercise, breathing practices, and sunshine are not usually thought of as medical treatments by the modern medical system. However, these can all be successfully used in the treatment of illness and more importantly, in the prevention of illness. For those of us who want to take responsibility for our own health, this book, containing natural remedies, can help. Most of the special materials that we use are found in the natural foods kitchen.

Macrobiotics itself is not a static, unchanging thing; it is a way of life that includes all the principles of vibrant health. These principles offer a unifying way to look at nature, a way to see the universe as a whole. To practice macrobiotics is to observe nature and apply what we learn to our lifestyles. This includes both our daily eating and our outlook on life. Our way of eating has an essential influence on our life experience. Macrobiotic dietary principles take into account differing needs according to climate, geography, age, sex, and level of activity. Tradition and intuition should guide us in our food choices as well as our life choices.

The following basic macrobiotic principles can act as a guide. Chances are if you remember these points, no obstacle will be too great for you. (See next page.)

YIN & YANG

Macrobiotics emphasizes the existence of a unifying principle. In short, it makes us aware of the unity in Life. The unifying

Basic Macrobiotic Principles

Health is the natural condition of human beings. It is our birthright.

Illness and unhappiness are unnatural conditions.

Health or sickness is not an accident or something inexplicable.

Sickness arises from how we live as a result of our own actions and thoughts.

Food is one of the very important factors in determining sickness.

We should eat seasonal foods that grow in our environment.

principle is thought to be the origin of all the opposites that exist. It is interesting isn't it, that from the unchanging comes the opposing forces which can change everything? These two opposing forces were called *Yin* and *Yang* by the ancient Chinese. These powerful tendencies create and destroy everything in this universe. Understanding the movement of change can be useful in establishing balance and creating health.

In our lives, when we have difficulty, we simply need to look at how we are encouraging such an imbalance. The realms of thinking, breathing, movement, diet, sleep, and sex—the six fundamental areas of life which contribute to our current state of health—are as far as we have to look. Anytime an imbalance is present, we have helped to create it. Our goal, then, is to prevent imbalances and to remedy any that may already be present. The body doesn't lie. By watching the body, its structure, movement and gestures, we can perceive balance or imbalance. All ancient medical systems were primarily concerned with observing and treating imbalance. In traditional Chinese healing practices the Yin/Yang principle was used. Basic to the understanding of this principle is the assumption that the elements of nature are temporary and changing. Recognizing this, human beings who want to follow nature must conduct their lives accordingly; that is, they must be prepared to adapt and change. These two forces are always opposite and antagonistic, and yet, at the same time, they are complementary, for they are always combining and cooperating. These two tendencies, constantly interacting, were understood in ancient China to create balance. This happens both inside the body and outside in the world. Simply stated, any illness is an imbalance of Yin and Yang.

With the predominance of one tendency giving way to the dominance of its opposite, and vice versa, everything therefore is constantly changing. Although always changing, each thing still contains both *yin* and *yang*. This fact creates a wholeness that is constantly evolving. Bound together, *yin* and *yang* unify. Yang is the inward movement that creates contraction. Yin is the outward movement that creates expansion. The following chart will give you an idea of Yin and Yang qualities.

The development of clear intuition is an aim of macrobiotics. Traditional wisdom tells us that the body and mind are not separate. With the application of macrobiotics, thinking, naturally becomes clearer. Judgment automatically improves. Our brain and mind begin to follow natural patterns, thereby not wasting energy with needless worry or preoccupations. Naturally, and with humility, wisdom develops.

When investigating the cause of illness, don't look for complicated reasons why you are not healthy. Look at the obvious. Pay attention to the following day to day activities: thinking, breathing, movement, diet, sex, and sleep. These are the fundamentals of health. Whenever there is a health problem, it can be found within one or more of these realms. If we are healthy, it is because we are following nature's way in each of these activities.

	More Yin ▼	More Yang ▲
Everyday Observations	rest	action
	dark	light
	moon	sun
	cold	hot
	large	small
	up	down
Body Structure	front of body or head	back of body or head
	soft parts	hard parts
	expanded organs	compacted organs
Body Location	peripheral parts	inner parts
	upper position (e.g., head)	lower position (e.g., legs)
Function	nervous function	digestive function
	female function	male function
	mental activities	physical activities
	eliminating function	consuming function
	ascending movement	descending movement
	expanding movement	contracting movement
	exhaling function (relaxation)	inhaling function (tension)
	physically inhaling (expansion)	physically exhaling (contraction)
	flexible	inflexible
	slow	rapid

Phases of the Moon

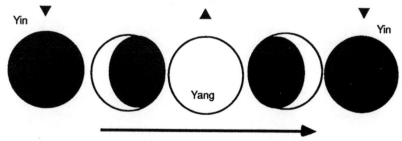

The movement of the moon cycle is an example of Yin/Yang movement.
One phase changing to another continually.

Natural Forces

For hundreds of thousands of years, our planet and all of its inhabitants have been affected by earthly and universal forces. It is the interaction of these common forces that has created the planet that we know. The sun's warmth, energy, and vibrations is vital to our existence. Its heat, interacting with moisture and vegetable seed, creates the plants and vegetables that serve as our food and shelter, and therefore ensure our survival. Water moistens the earth, keeping it green. The elements in water feed the plants which, in their growing process, give us oxygen, an important part of the air that we breathe. The abundant air that is so essential to all animal life is another universal force which is inter-related with the sun and water. All of these forces, plus vibrations from the stars, planets, and space beyond this planet, have formed our world.

Without these universal forces, life would be very different; we would be unable to survive. Survival is dependent on something that is beyond us as individuals. It is nature that nurtures and cares for both plant and animal life. This wisdom has fascinated human beings since earliest times. Ancient people had reverence and curiosity regarding these powers. Their culture, way of life, religion, agriculture, and medicine reflected this keen interest. Works of art, poetry, and handiwork remain as reminders of their reverence for these forces. They understood that nature controlled everything. Weather and crop success was in the hands of nature. When the harvest was abundant, they knew that nature could be generous. When crops failed by drought or other natural disasters, they knew that it could be extremely severe.

To a large degree, our present society has forgotten the power of nature. We have forgotten that it is the source of life. Our modern way of living artificially insulates us from these forces. Our cities are frequently empty of trees, flowers, and grass. Except for rare city parks, we see and feel only concrete, glass, plastic, and other artificial materials. Our clothing, more and more, comes from synthetic fabric. Our food is often less then natural and whole. Most restaurant food as well as homestyle cooking consists of refined foodstuffs containing artificial flavors and chemicals.

The belief that man-made science is superior to natural order is presently popular worldwide. In the past, ancient people trusted in the gods; today we put our trust in science and technology. We hope, like our predecessors, that the never-ending problems of life and survival can be answered.

Science has become an important part of modern life. However, problems arise when we forget that nature exists independently, and science is only a part of nature. Without nature, science cannot exist. Without science, nature still exists. This point must remain clear if we are to find accurate and permanent solutions to our problems.

The force of nature is in every one of us. It is in all things that exist. We should look to nature for our direction. If we go along with nature, we go along with the larger forces that helped to create us. If we fail to follow the way of nature, we can expect problems and unhappiness. Goethe expressed the idea thus: "Nature understands no jesting; she is always true, always serious, always severe; she is always right, and the errors and faults are always those of man. The man incapable of appreciating her, she despises; and only to the apt, the pure, and the true, does she resign herself, and reveal her secrets."

Traditional Chinese medicine is based on natural laws. Thousands of years ago, a medical system evolved which patterned itself on the observations of nature. It was realized that everything was constantly changing. The changes were predictable and from

this came the laws of *Yin* and *Yang*, the governing forces within the universe. The ancients saw that energy circulated in a distinct pattern from organ to organ within the body—much as a river flows, within its banks, on its voyage from mountain to sea. This vital energy moved from organ to organ, animating each one, giving each organ the fuel to function. We know this as the "meridian" or "channel" system.

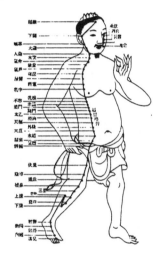

Any obstruction of this flow in vital energy created problems. In order to cure the problem, balance had to be reestablished. But the cure must be governed by natural law.

Looking outward to our immediate surroundings puts us into direct contact with natural order. When you sit by a river in the warmth of a summer day, you feel the comfort and openness that is part of this segment of nature's yearly cycle. In the cold winter winds, you feel the chilling aspect of nature's cycle. One season makes you feel warm, relaxed, and comfortable while another season can make you feel cold, tight, and somewhat rigid. Each one of the seasons has an effect on us and makes us become like that season.

Looking inwardly at ourselves we can see very clearly the natural order that exists., You don't have to read textbooks or have teachers explain to you what is natural and what is not. Our own biological and emotional needs and urges are natural order. These are, themselves, natural forces. When you are hungry or thirsty, this is nature speaking to you. When you have to go to the toilet, this is nature talking to you. The urge to make love and have a family and children are absolutely natural forces that need no instructions. The social need to share with friends and laugh together is part of being human. To deny these urges is to deny nature and to violate her laws.

Clearly natural forces have created us and continue to work within us. Our human experiences serve as reminders to let us know if we are living within the natural order or not. By observing natural laws, we can learn to correct and eliminate many of our problems. For example, in nature, animals eat their food whole. We should follow this example. Our "daily bread" should be whole grains, not refined flour. In the same way, our actions should be complete, not fragmented. As nature completes a cycle, moving from one season to the next, we human beings should complete our cycles by finishing the things we set out to do. If we follow natural order, our physical and mental health is more secured then if we do not follow. If wrong living habits are continued long enough they will develop into troubles. Nature demonstrates that life is to be lived simply. Illness is an expression of our ignorance of these forces. Given the uncertainty and complexity of modern life, it is still up to us to decide how to live.

Cause of Illness

From the moment of conception within a mother's womb, we are living, moving, and growing creatures. This energy of life comes partly from our parents as genetic inheritance and partly from the nourishment of food, drink, emotions, ideas, and vibrations. Because we are alive, we must keep ourselves in good condition. Without this constant conditioning, it is easy to deteriorate. At times we say to ourselves that we don't feel well. At that moment, we already know that something is going wrong. This feeling is our signal that normal body functions are beginning to make changes. The unpleasant symptoms of the aches and pains are an attempt by the body to reestablish harmony. But, to you, that headache certainly doesn't feel like harmony!

When symptoms are present, the energy within the internal organs as well as the muscles and tissues doesn't circulate well. Physical and emotional suffering is an expression of imbalance. These changes are, nonetheless, the body's attempt to conserve life energy and promote long-term health.

The cause of illness was recorded in ancient medical textbooks thousands of years ago in China and India—imbalance. For example when the heart becomes imbalanced we may see either high or low blood pressure. When the pancreas is affected, the result is often hypoglycemia (low blood sugar) or diabetes (high blood sugar). When we don't feel well, it can be a single organ or many body systems that act out of harmony with the rest.

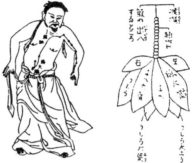

Ancient illustrations of
Lung and Lung meridian.

Human beings belong to nature. If we follow the way of nature, we aren't supposed to get many problems. Why do we get sick? If humans are superior, why do so many have such serious problems? Without knowing it, many of us live our lives out of harmony with nature. When our lifestyle, which includes all the things that we do throughout the day, does not go along with the way nature intended, difficulties arise. In order to correct this situation, we must find out what it is in our daily life that is inappropriate. Where have we created our greatest imbalance? How have we violated natural law?

"The Cause of All Illness is an Imbalance of Yin and Yang."
—Gong Bai, M.D.
Neuro-surgeon, Shanghai, People's Republic of China

Once an illness or imbalance is there , we all want to get rid of it, don't we? Already, even on a subconscious level, we are trying to make a new balance. Because of our illness, we become very busy trying to cure it. We may go from doctor to doctor asking advice and, without realizing it, spending a lot of time on ourselves. We have no time for others because we are so preoccupied with our own troubles. Our mentality begins to change as we become self-centered. At this point not only is the body ill, but the mind also becomes sick.

We are made up of trillions of cells. They are affected very easily by the condition of the fluids which are both inside and around all body cells. If these body fluids become closer to an acidic condition, then dysfunction rapidly occurs within each cell and the organs that are made of these cells. Hyperactive, underactive or dead nerve cells can dramatically change the function of the entire body. Many scientific studies have shown the importance of a healthy autonomic nervous system. Imbalance between the sympathetic branch (which governs daytime activity) and the parasympathetic branch (which governs nighttime and healing activity) is the cause for many of the common problems we see today. This nervous system imbalance can affect all cells and organs within the body. An imbalance at the cellular level affects the whole organism. When we eat inappropriate foods, such as sugar or fat, or when breathing is shallow and superficial, the possibility of imbalances occurring becomes very great. When imbalances occur, we must discover their sources—this is easier then you might think. The source for most degenerative illness is what we do or don't do day to day. A quick check of how we eat, breathe, move, think, and handle stress will show us our mistakes.

After we begin to regain our health, it becomes obvious that we are in a more balanced state. Our symptoms decrease and eventually go away. At the same time, our interest is not only in ourselves, but we begin to think about others. If we can maintain this balanced state, even with minor ups and downs, an excess of energy will accumulate that we can use to help our families and friends. How to maintain this balance is an aim of life.

There is an old Chinese proverb which gives us something to think about: "Unless you change direction, you are likely to arrive where you are headed."

Fundamentals of Health

Although we may think that abundant vitality and good health should be our birthright, we soon discover that this is rarely true. Being in good health and maintaining that state take constant attention and diligent work. We can all think of someone close to us who suffers from some chronic or serious illness. We wonder, is it something that s/he did or didn't do that has created such a condition? What are the factors that can prevent illness and promote health?

Genetic inheritance, education, and job activities throughout life build not only one's character, but also one's body. Food, drink, emotions, stress, and what we think add to the body chemistry and make us who we are. We are a combination of our family genetics and environment.

In adddition to our family heritage and growth environment, the things that we do throughout the day are extremely important in helping to shape our wellness picture. These day-to-day activities can be considered our fundamentals of health. These aspects of living are the cornerstones upon which our health and vitality rests. If we care for the foundation, all which is built upon it will withstand the storms of life. It is the little everyday things in life that are important and have the possibility of bringing the greatest happiness.

Carefully observe your activities of thinking, breathing, movement, diet, sex, and sleep, for these are the six fundamentals of health. Within this realm lies success or failure in your physical health and emotional happiness.

Consciousness

All body functions and thoughts are controlled by the brain. It serves as the central control office. Located in the head, which is the uppermost or most yin part of the body, the brain function coordinates all physical movement, thinking, and emotions. All body parts are affected by its condition. Likewise, the condition of the body has an effect on the brain. We know that nourishment from food creates blood. The quality of our blood influences the quality of our thinking. The brain and body are inseparable, but it is the brain that determines the direction of the rest of the body.

Messages from the brain to the body and from the body to the brain pass through the neck. It is the neck that acts as the connection. It is important that the neck is flexible, relaxed and in proper condition.

Our sense organs can be considered receptors of stimuli from the external environment. They transmit the messages they receive to the brain and the energy channel system within the body (see energy chart, page 122). The brain's function is to sort, store, and send the messages it receives. Oriental medicine states that every part of the body communicates with other parts through the channel system (see energy chart, page 122). Because of this connection, emotions produced in the brain in response to various stimuli, can be responsible for disturbing the function of any part of the body. The emotions of anger, fear, worry, excitability, depression, anxiety, joy, etc. have definite effects on the rest of the body. The example of the worried person who develops stomach ulcers is all too plain. If an imbalance of yin and yang exists in either the brain and/or body, a problem will develop. Excessive emotion takes its toll on the body.

The physical brain influences thinking and judgment. The ancient memory of our heritage, as well as the current, immediate learned memory is influenced by the condition and the quality of the brain. Our will, sense of direction, and happiness are the totality of the function of the body, mind, and spirit. If our thinking is to be truly clear and accurate, we can not overlook the brain. Because we think and reason, we are different from other animals—it is our thinking which guides us in life.

Breathing

Breathing is an important part of maintaining vibrant health. It is the most important ingredient for our nutrition. We get proteins, vitamins, carbohydrates, and fats from food, but without the air that we breathe, we would not get much value from the foods that we eat. Without the oxygen that is in air, food will not energize our bodies, just as fire without air, will not burn. Oxygen combines with the carbon and hydrogen furnished by food. These reactions generate heat and provide the living organism with energy for physical work, as well as for the many other processes essential for life, such as digestion, growth, and brain function. Breathing exhales carbon dioxide, which if not eliminated, builds up in the body, causing the tissue fluids to be too acid. In order to live, we must breathe—but what kind of breathing patterns do you have?

Have you ever noticed that when you are absorbed in the suspense or drama of a film you find yourself holding your breath? Or when you become angry, your breathing is shallow, coming only from your chest? Rapid breathing is a signal that something is wrong; both your physical and mental powers are weak at this time.

Deep breathing is the best way to maintain health. A long, deep, full inhalation and exhalation will expand and contract the lungs. These two opposite motions make a balanced breathing rhythm. The breath is a combination of yin and yang forces in cooperation. It is the balance of the autonomic nervous system with the sympathetic and parasympathetic branches which affects the functions of the internal organs. It is breathing, to a large degree, which affects the nervous system and therefore the functioning of all the other internal organs. Breathing affects the quality of blood through digestion and assimilation. Abdominal breathing and exhalation are connected with blood circulation. The long, deep, rhythmical breath supplies both essential oxygen to body cells and also mental stability. Only when the breath is calm can the mind be calm.

Inhalation expands the lungs creating a degree of tension within the body. This activates the nervous system. Our exhalation contracts the lungs, thereby relaxing nerve activity and loosening a tense body. Holding your breath makes for mental concentration and forceful body movement but at the same time it can create rigidity . If you feel tense often, emphasize your exhalation more— consciously make it a little longer than the inhalation. Make it longer and stronger. You can do this at any time. If you can control your breathing you can become really free.

The daily practice of breathing exercises will improve overall well-being. Try to spend some time practicing each day. Practice deep breathing while walking and working. However, first of all, become consciously aware of your breathing by practicing the following exercise. You can then integrate this correct breathing into your daily life.

Sit with your back straight either in a chair or on the floor with your legs crossed in any posture that is comfortable. Relax your thinking and let the thoughts just drift off. Let your shoulders, then your arms, neck, and head become relaxed. Keep your eyes only half open with your gaze about five feet in front of you on the floor. Breathe only through your nose. Make your inhalation and exhalation the same length. Mentally, you can feel your whole body breathing, not just the nose and lungs. Practice this for as long as you like, up to twenty minutes at a time.

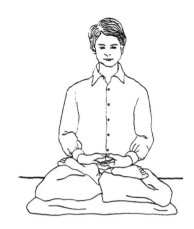

We cannot live without air for more than four minutes. With deep breathing, we get over seven times the normal volume of oxygen. This means that we enrich the blood with oxygen and vitality, which, in turn, brings even more energy and essential life force. In the case of cancer, cancer cells do not like oxygen. They thrive in an unclean environment. Cancer patients feel much better when they combine proper diet, breathing, exercise, and physical movement. Even if they do only a little, there are positive effects . The richness of the blood is the basis of the entire body's health, and the blood can be called rich only if it contains the necessary amount of oxygen and other nutrients. This comes from proper breathing, whole natural foods, and exercise.

Movement

Our bodies are made to move and be active. From birth until death, this process goes on. Modern people don't physically move as often as in the past. Formerly the majority of people worked on the farm, which is physically very demanding. Walking, bending, and lifting are activities that were a natural part of the farm day.

With technology, very few people are required to do strenuous work. It looks as though we will be required to do even less in the future. Office work uses the brain but leaves the body sedentary for many hours each day. This lack of movement creates many problems including circulatory problems and weak, atrophied muscles. Ancient peoples had to work hard to forage for food—it wasn't so easy to get. They were active in obtaining the food and, as it wasn't so abundant, they ate less. Wild animals also must expend energy through stalking and hunting to feed themselves. We, on the other hand, have very little difficulty in obtaining food. We can go to the market, restaurant or coffeeshop anytime we want. We eat too much and don't walk enough.

On the other hand, exercise is becoming a national pastime. There is a growing interest in jogging, tennis, aerobic activity, dance classes, etc. With this recent upsurge of physical activity come warnings from the medical community that exercise can be dangerous to your health. Many Americans have been somewhat lazy in doing physical activity in the past and, just as they start a physical health program, they are warned that exercise can be just as dangerous as their previous sedentary ways. How can we make sense from this? Should we exercise? Let's look at some of the recent facts concerning exercise and health.

Those who favor exercise say that its greatest benefit is that it can prevent heart and vessel disease, the number one killer in the

U.S. But is that true? The answer is not clear-cut. Formerly it was thought that exercise could lower cholesterol levels (a material which blocks the blood passages, especially those in the heart). It was also thought that it could lower blood pressure, whereas actually, while exercising, your blood pressure increases! It has been found that regular exercise does not lower the cholesterol levels in the blood. However, it does raise the level of high density lipoprotein (HDL), which is considered "good cholesterol." Studies have shown that people with higher levels of HDL have a lower risk of heart disease. Exercise raises the levels of HDL. Therefore, physically active people are less likely to have heart disease.

This good news, however, is a statement based on averages and does not apply to each individual. Further tests have demonstrated that for those with existing heart disease, the chances of having a heart attack while exercising are seven times greater than if they sat in a chair and never moved. Should we never exercise because of the fear of dropping dead during our "health" program? Studies concluded that the temporary risk during exercise does not outweigh the long-term benefits. Therefore, it is better to exercise—but if you are out of shape, use caution at first.

When beginning an exercise program, you should take care and use common sense so as not to overexert yourself. You can easily include movement in your daily life rather then relying on extra routines: walk rather then drive, reach, bend or stretch while playing with the children or doing the housework. If there is a history of heart disease in the family, if you have a personal history of heart trouble, or if you are over thirty-five years old and have been sedentary for some time, then care should be taken before you start exercising. Medical authorities suggest that these groups should have a stress test taken before they begin an exercise program.

Once you begin an exercise program, you should be alert to

some warning signs. Pain in the chest, throat, arms, pit of the stomach, or shoulder and neck areas, that comes on during exercise, is a warning sign that you may be pushing your limit. These pains may indicate that there is blockage in the vessels of the heart.

Running fifteen miles per week is the maximum distance necessary to strengthen the heart. Jogging more than fifteen miles per week doesn't do the heart any more good. On the contrary, it tears down the knees and joints and puts unnecessary stress on the heart vessels, perhaps even setting you up for a heart attack. You only have to do so much exercise to strengthen and benefit the cardiovascular system. To qualify as beneficial, the exercise must involve the large muscles, such as the arms, legs, or trunk; it must be nonstop for twenty-five to thirty minutes; and it must be repeated three to five times per week.

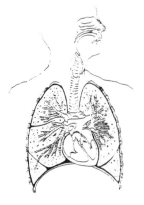

The joints, bones, and muscles are responsible for the initiation of movement. In order to sustain a movement, we must have a strong breathing capacity. Lung capacity and circulation ability increase naturally with use. To develop coordination though, one must exercise.

Other kinds of exercise such as yoga and Do-In (a form of self-massage), systematically coordinate the body, breath, mind, and spirit. They are also important in teaching economic use of energy. They improve posture, which significantly affects not only the nerves, but also every major system in the body. A balanced program of exercise, including some rigorous action and some controlled stretching, is very helpful.

Diet

Diet is perhaps the most personal of all the fundamentals of health. Specific foods have certain connections for us with family, holidays, and good and bad times in our lives. This adds up to making our eating habits difficult ones to change. Usually it is only illness that causes people to begin to consider alternatives to current food consumption trends. Changing your diet is a bigger adjustment than one might at first realize, but it certainly can be enjoyable. In fact, this modification can be one of the most profound and exciting adventures of your life. Not only do the benefits of increased strength and vitality make a change in eating worthwhile, but savings in food bills and medical costs are notable advantages as well.

Common sense tells us that we should eat smaller portions and eliminate junk food if we are serious about maintaining vibrant health and preventing illness. But what else should be done? Did you know that agriculture has changed dramatically since the end of World War II? At that time, the actively growing oil industry decided to develop a new market for their products. This market was agriculture. In the 1950's, chemical and petroleum products began to be used in the growth and processing of our basic foods. These were used as toxic sprays to kill insects and as artificial fertilizers. At the same time chemical and petroleum products began to be used in the hybridization process of plant seeds. With chemicals, new strains of plants were developed. Furthermore, for a variety of reasons—generally to make marketing easier—extensive processing and the refinement of foods was actively pursued. From the view of nature, all of these processes weaken and devitalize the original food, changing it to something unrecognizable as far as nutrient content and taste are concerned.

To counter this growing trend in agriculture, our food choices should be local and in-season varieties of organically grown, whole natural foods, whenever possible. It is best to minimize or avoid refined, processed, and commercially canned foods. If we adhere to the traditional advice of eating only whole foods, one can see the difficulty of eating certain foods such as a cow or pig—we would have to eat from head to tail! To eat food in its entirety satisfies the conditions necessary for living. It is easy to accomplish this when using vegetables. Even with sophisticated laboratory technology it is impossible to isolate all the vitamins and minerals necessary for life. However, eating a balanced diet of whole foods, which are natural sources of all vitamins and minerals, assures us of all our requirements.

Confirming the macrobiotic view, a growing body of medical evidence points to seed foods as a significant protection from disease. The National Academy of Science has stated that the incidence of breast cancer, colon cancer and prostate cancer could be cut substantially if Americans ate more "seed foods." Other scientific studies corroborate these findings. Seed foods include all whole grains such as whole wheat, brown rice, and barley; beans such as kidney, lentils, and chickpeas; and commonly known seeds such as sesame, sunflower, and pumpkin. Studies have shown that seed foods contain protease inhibitors which appear to have a protective, anti-cancer effect.

Sugar, chemicals, preservatives, additives, and colorings can be considered poisonous foods and will break down the body. Building a house takes time, while the opposite process—tearing it down—happens quickly. To build health takes consistent attention, while it is so easy to lose. For example, chemicals used in agriculture, food processing, and food preparation are sure to create imbalances in the immune system when eaten regularly. These can easily be avoided if you are eating whole, organically grown food, just as nature made it—complete with all the vitamins, minerals, enzymes, and fiber—without a trace of artificial color, preservatives, or flavors. You can taste the difference!

Food can be divided into two categories; they are those to avoid and those to emphasize in the diet. The first group includes refined foods such as white flour and sugar. The second group includes vegetables and fruits. These should be grown in the climate in which you live. Temperate zone people, as in the U.S. and Europe, should be eating carrots, cauliflower, turnips, kale, onions, squash, garbanzo beans, apples, pears, strawberries, etc., and not bananas, papayas, etc.which are tropical in origin and therefore not suitable for people living in temperate climates.

Animal proteins like beef, chicken, pork, eggs, etc., as well as all forms of dairy products (milk, cream, butter, cheese, cottage cheese, ice cream, yogurt and kefir), should be minimized. The high fat content, as well as the antibiotics that the animal has received, are injurious to humans.

In addition to the animal fats found in beef and butter, other forms of fat are best avoided. These include lard, shortening, and margarine. Poor-quality blended or refined oils should not be used. These fatty items create a stickiness which causes red blood cells to lump together. Clumps of cells have less surface area than individual cells and therefore, less opportunity to carry oxygen and nutrients to the body's internal organs. A common symptom of sticky blood is fatigue.

Artificial foods should be avoided. This includes the flavoring, coloring, and preserving agents that are in all instant foods. Artificial sweeteners, as well as sugar, brown sugar, turbinado sugar, honey, molasses, and corn syrup, should be avoided.

Alcoholic beverage consumption should be limited and

occasional. Soft drinks and artificially sweetened juices and drinks should be completely avoided. Care should be taken with the use of stimulating teas and coffee.

Foods recommended in the macrobiotic diet encompass a wide variety of textures and tastes. Variety in your choices should bring complete satisfaction in your eating. Delicious dishes can be prepared using the ingredients listed below.

Whole grains are the most important foods in a macrobiotic diet. Also included are beans, roots, round vegetables such as pumpkin and squash, and hardy, green leafy vegetables. Soups, nuts, seeds, seaweeds, fruits and fish are also included.

Whole grains: whole wheat, millet, brown rice, rye, barley, oats, buckwheat, and corn. These can be used in their whole form or as flour in foods such as breads, tortillas, chapatis and noodles.

Vegetables: brussel sprouts, kale, watercress, mustard and collard greens, chinese cabbage, red and green cabbage, bok choy and sprouts, string beans, broccoli, cauliflower, beans (e.g., lentils, garbanzo, navy, pinto, aduki, and black), winter squash, pumpkins, acorn and buttercup squash, leeks, scallions, onions, turnips, carrots, rutabagas.

Soup: miso, tamari, vegetable, or bean soups.

Seaweeds: dulse, nori, wakame, kombu, arame, hijiki, agar, Irish moss and sea palm.

Fruits: apples, cherries, pears, strawberries, chestnuts, berries, etc.

Nuts: walnuts, almonds, hazelnuts, etc.

Seeds: pumpkin, sunflower, sesame, squash.

Fish: sole, snapper, cod, trout, and other white meat fish.

Beverages: non-stimulating teas such as twig, barley, toasted brown rice and corn, mild herbal teas, vegetable and fruit juices.

After a period of eating well, we begin to understand our physical and emotional needs. This process develops naturally, if the lifestyle is relatively balanced. This understanding is known as intuition.

The following guidelines will aid in the development of the intuitive process.

Eat When Hungry, Drink When Thirsty. If we eat or drink too much or when the body has no need for food or drink, then we are not responding to our inner voice. Instead, we are indulging our sensorial appetite. Overindulgence in anything is harmful to one's well-being.

Choose and Eat Only Natural Whole Foods. Use whole, unrefined foods as much as possible. Choose vegetables that are fresh and chemical-free. Avoid processed, canned, and frozen foods. Vegetables from the sea are rich in minerals and are very healthful.

Chew Well. Good food tastes better the more you chew. Brown rice, for example, becomes sweeter when chewed well, whereas meat quickly loses its flavor. In this way, chewing also helps you distinguish between good and bad food. When you are sick, chewing well is essential. Digestion of complex carbohydrates begins in the mouth—so the more you chew, the better absorption and assimilation you'll have. To develop spirituality and sensitivity, it is also necessary to chew well. Mental clarity and judgment improve with mastication. Also, complete chewing leads to satisfaction after a meal, and lessens the desire to overeat. Chewing well does not mean chewing slowly! One who chews well should finish the meal along with everyone else.

Eat Only to Eighty Percent Capacity. Never eat until you are full. Overeating creates excess, which, if it is not discharged, will cause imbalance. Overeating clouds the mind, makes you feel sleepy, and hinders your capacity to be active. A person who eats only to eighty percent capacity has a greater chance of success.

Enjoy Your Meals. All food should be eaten with the spirit of gratitude and enjoyment. Cooking, which is an art, and the presentation and consumption of the food should be a joyful experience. It can be one of life's greatest pleasures.

Do Not Eat When Upset. If you are very tired, do not eat. If you are having emotional difficulties, do not eat. At these times, the body is not prepared to receive food or to digest it properly. Take a walk to calm down before you eat.

Your Kitchen Is Your Pharmacy. Our daily food is our medicine. Thus, the proper selection and preparation of daily meals is essential to the maintenance of health. Most illness, then, can be avoided with proper nutrition. Studies say that seventy percent of illness is diet-related. The importance of cooking cannot be overstated. Good macrobiotic cookbooks and cooking classes are essential in mastering the art of healthy food preparation.

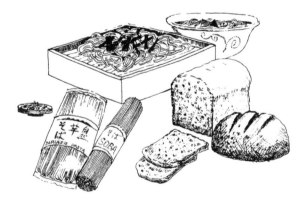

Properties of Specific Whole Grains

Corn: most fruitlike of the grains; cooling; moisturizing; nourishing to the heart and circulatory system; encourages healthy teeth.

Oats: soothing and restorative to the nervous system; valuable in relieving insomnia; helps normalize thyroid function; strengthens cardiac muscle; helps relieve constipation; used as a poultice for relief of itching or to heal and beautify the skin.

Barley: strengthens and builds blood; easily digested; treats diarrhea; reduces   fever and internal heat; dissolves tumors; good for cancer, especially pearl barley (hato mugi); soothes inflamed membranes.

Brown Rice: high in B vitamins; beneficial to the lungs; beneficial for diabetics; when eaten raw can expel worms.

Millet: an alkaline grain; warming; beneficial to the stomach, pancreas and spleen; beneficial for diabetics; helps prevent miscarriage.

Wheat: encourages fat formation; promotes clear thinking; beneficial to the liver.

Rye: increases strength and endurance; aids muscle formation; warming; aids fingernail, hair and bone growth; contains fluorine for tooth enamel strength.

Buckwheat: warming and drying; increases circulation to both feet and hands; builds blood; source of vitamin E; high in protein.

Sex

From observing nature it is evident that all animals indulge in the sexual act as a matter of reproduction. It is necessary for the continuation of the species. So from a universal perspective, reproduction is the inate, animal purpose of sex.

Another function of sex is pleasure. Intimacy with others is an important part of life. It feels good and makes us happy. Problems arise when people over emphasize sexual gratification and make the personal pleasure of sexual intercourse their only goal at the expense of relationship, commitment, and communication.

This over emphasis comes from many sources. One obvious cause is the overconsumption of animal protein. The eating of beef, chicken, eggs, and other animal foods can create over-stimulation of the sexual organs, as can overeating of any food. This stimulation encourages sexual preoccupation and abnormal sexual tendencies. This may be displayed as an act of adult sexual violence or physical, emotional, or sexual abuse of children.

In the 1600's in Japan, *Yojokun, the Secret of Health Preservation,* was written by Ekiken Kaibara. In this book much is written about the art of long life and the role of sex.

Although we may disagree with what Ekiken says, it is interesting to consider what was written over three hundred years ago. "At twenty years of age people should have a sexual discharge no more than once in a period of four days, at thirty once in eight days, at forty once in sixteen days, and at fifty once in twenty days. At sixty a person should no longer discharge his energy sexually unless he is particularly vigorous physically, in which case he can do so once a month. However, if a person who is extremely vigorous and healthy suppresses the urge too long, this can cause trouble. If a person allows sexual desire to get the better of him, sexual gratification will become a bad habit that will be hard to break." In other words too much sex as well as not enough can cause trouble.

If you are in a good, healthy condition, then proper sexual behavior will take care of itself.

Sleep

One of the most natural and enjoyable activities that we all do is sleep. Sleep is that period of inactivity where we are unaware and generally unresponsive to our environment. Certain body changes occur during sleep. Sleep itself has two phases. The first phase is the period of nonrapid eye movement. During this time the heart and respiratory rates slow down, the muscles are greatly but not completely relaxed, and the eyelids remain quite still.

During the second phase, rapid eye movement sleep (REM), the eyeballs move jerkily under closed lids, the heart and breathing rates quicken, and the muscles (especially the neck muscles) completely relax. This is the stage where dreams occur.

Although most people experience this dreaming period, it is not a sign of good health. It is a working function, not one of rest. During sleep the body and mind should be in a resting state. Healthy people do not normally dream. Dreaming is the body's way of processing either physical or psychological residues. If, during the day, emotional snags are dealt with completely, there will be no residue that needs to be processed during sleep. In a similar way, when no agitating materials are circulating in the brain (such as fats, sugar, beef, coffee and chemical stimulants), no pictures or dreams will be perceived. However, true dreams can occur for healthy people, which can serve as predictions of things to come or contact with spiritual vibrations.

If you are eating properly and exercising, then the recovery time for your organs and systems occurs quickly. This means that a healthy body sleeps less. Not eating three hours before bed-time will promote sound sleep. In addition to a shorter sleeping time, a healthy person has very deep sleep, the body is soft and the breathing slow. During sleep there should be very little body movement. Movement during sleep is a corrective mechanism by the body. If there are imbalances, the body will make adjustments to try to correct and eliminate these abnormal conditions while you sleep. A healthy sleeping posture is flat on the back with the arms relaxed at the sides. Generally, sleeping on the sides or on the stomach shows troubles.

Sleep is very much like death except that breathing and vital organ functions continue at a minimum rate. It is during sleep that the body's self-healing mechanism functions. It is during this time when new cells are constructed and old cells recycled.

Ideally, when you awake from sleep, you should feel happy and clear-headed. You should have positive thoughts and an optimistic attitude. You should feel prepared to start another exciting day. A healthy person awakes alert without any aches or pains. The body should feel flexible and not stiff. Sleep is the great refresher and energizer.

Four Conditions of Sleep

1. When the body and mind are evenly tired, then sleep naturally comes quickly.

2. If you have done little activity and are not tired enough, then sleep won't come. Your body has no need of it.

3. When there is an imbalance between the body and the mind, normal sleep won't come. For example, when the brain is overworking from the artificial stimulation of coffee or other stimulants and/or you are worried and mentally concerned about something, the mind won't let you sleep even when the body is tired.

4. When physical troubles are present, especially a stiff painful neck or hips, natural sleep is difficult in coming.

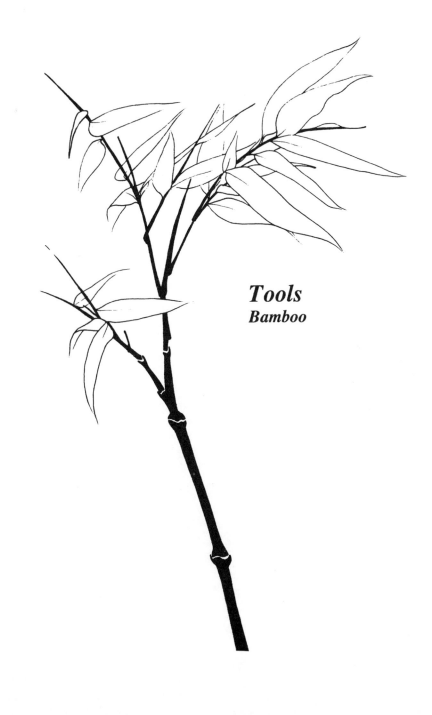

Tools
Bamboo

Preparation for Treatment

Administered professionally or within the family, shiatsu is
more than a medical treatment. It can link us with those we love. It
is very effective in relaxing people, thereby creating a feeling of to-
getherness and peace. This family treatment, while being comfortable, is still effective in dealing with specific problems. One of the
aims of shiatsu is to maintain balance for both giver and receiver.
That is, the effect of both giving and receiving a treatment makes
you feel more centered, more like yourself. It makes you feel whole
and connected to the earth and to life. A treatment should not be done
in a casual way, for example, as a preliminary to sex.

Here are several suggestions for both the giver and the
receiver of the treatment which will enhance both the enjoyment and
effectivenes of the session. Not only should the receiver benefit from
the session, the giver must also profit. For the giver, a successful
treatment can be done only when sufficient energy is in reserve to
be given away. This means that the giver must be in a state of good
health. If the giver is fatigued or weak, the session will be unsatis-
factory. The combination of proper eating, correct breathing, and
adequate day to day movement will ensure the vitality necessary for
good treatments. If the giver is eating too much meat, eggs, fish, and

cheese, then his or her attitude can be tight and aggressive. It will be difficult to honestly listen to the problems of others whom s/he is treating. The treatment itself can be given too roughly, thereby making the receiver feel uncomfortable. If sugar, oil, chemicals, or other artificial foods are eaten the giver can easily become distracted, losing the ability to concentrate. The giver won't be able to focus on the treatment and can easily become depressed and negative.

Advice to the Giver

Cleanliness

Before using your hands and feet as tools of treatment, be sure that they are washed and clean. The fingernails should be cut short so as not to hurt the receiver.

Concentration

In order to center yourself, which will allow a greater focusing power, some time of meditation or controlled breathing exercise should be performed before you begin the treatment. This can be done at the beginning of each day.

Attention to Breathing

Your own breath should be rhythmic, deep, and slow. Breathing should come from the diaphragm. This will minimize fatigue as well as maintain mental clarity. Your attention should also be on the breathing pattern of the receiver; watch his or her breath. A coordinated breath, where both the giver and receiver are breathing together, greatly increases the treatment's effectiveness. This type of breathing promotes relaxation especially for the receiver. If the receiver's breathing rate becomes too fast, you can adjust the treatment to slow it down to a relaxed rate. Tell the receiver to breath in deeply and then give the command to breath out. You can set the pace.

Clothing

For greatest flexibility of movement and for comfort, the giver should wear loose, cotton clothing. Natural fibers breath and allow better air circulation next to your body. Jewelry should be removed.

Posture

Your body position is important both for the success of the treatment and for your own good as well. The back should be straight and the hips and knees relaxed. Don't twist your body. If you become unbalanced, it is better to readjust yourself rather than stay in an uncomfortable position. When you lean over, as when you press the back, bend from the hips and not from the small of the back. Any hunched position puts stress on the vertebrae and nervous system. Most importantly, when you do a complete shiatsu follow a specific routine. This conserves your energy.

Rhythm

The body of the receiver is a fine instrument. As with a piano, the giver, if attentive, can learn to play and harmonize with the instrument. If the giver and receiver are breathing well together a natural rhythm can be established. When shiatsu is given with a sense of harmony, the receiver feels very good. If the rhythm is off or the giver is insensitive to the receiver, then the receiver won't feel so good when the session is finished.

Support

When treating any part of the body always be attentive to how it feels to the receiver. Make sure that they feel comfortable and secure. For example when rotating the head don't allow the shoulders to roll about. Stabilize the area that you are working on. You will then be able to successfully focus your treatment.

Stillness

The purpose of shiatsu is to use touch to create peace. Our direction in the session is to accomplish this goal. Don't argue during a treatment. Even further, it is best not to talk too much especially nonessential talk such as gossip.

Confidence

During shiatsu, and perhaps throughout our lives, if we have confidence in our action then we can be successful. If your condition is not good, or you are uncertain of your capability to treat someone's problem, then you better not try to do it. To be on the safe side, if you lack confidence do not treat the receiver.

Environment

Give shiatsu in a place that is quiet and as free from distraction as possible. The session can be done on clean, comfortable cushions or a blanket placed on the floor. A small natural fiber pillow can be used under the head.

After the Treatment

With the contact of shiatsu, there is an exchange of energy between the giver and receiver. Several simple methods can be used to clean the receiver's vibrations from your own after treatment. Vigorously shaking the hands or clapping them together several times will disperse the receiver's vibrations and clear the connection between you. Washing the hands is also effective.

Advice to the Receiver

Trust

When receiving a treatment, the body can relax very deeply where there is trust between the receiver and giver. If you can not trust the family member or friend who is about to give you shiatsu, perhaps it is best not to receive the treatment. Without your trust it is difficult for them to touch you.

Clothing

When preparing for shiatsu you should remove any jewelry and socks or stockings. Thin cotton clothing is best to wear during the session.

Cleanliness

In the home situation, perhaps a bath or shower can be taken before receiving shiatsu. This will relax the muscles. The warm water promotes better circulation as well.

Information

It is better to wait two hours after meals before receiving shiatsu. Prior to the session, tell the giver any information about your present condition that seems useful. If you have had any past back or knee injuries, briefly explain the details. Any current problems should also be voiced. This information allows the treatment to be adjusted to properly suit you.

Female Concerns

Shiatsu can be given during menstruation or pregnancy if there are no complicating factors. If a woman usually has excessive menstrual flow, it may be best to skip shiatsu during this time. If the expectant mother has had a history of miscarriage, it would also be best to avoid vigorous shiatsu. A light touch or laying on of hands would be appropriate.

Breathing

During the treatment, concentrate your breathing on the exhalation, especially when pressure is being given. Always coordinate your breathing with the giver so that you are inhaling and exhaling at the same time.

Rest

If possible, after the treatment, continue to lie down and rest for ten to fifteen minutes. This will bring better results from the shiatsu.

Confidence

Whether the shiatsu treatment is given by a friend, family member, or professional, have confidence that the session will help you. Learning to relax allows your natural healing ability to surface.

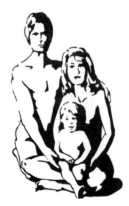

Shiatsu Technique

Our everyday observations can be useful in watching health changes of family members and friends. Usually you can tell when someone is suffering or unhappy. This simple recognition is the basis of diagnosis. We can easily be aware of many physical and emotional troubles just by being attentive.

The first feature to observe in others is the face. Posture, movement, gestures, and voice also tell us about how someone is feeling. Features of the face can confirm your analysis. Facial expression can be a very good indicator of emotion. Facial color is another obvious sign. For example, a pale, lifeless face indicates anemia and lack of energy, whereas a brilliantly red face can indicate high blood pressure or overconsumption of sugar, alcohol, or drugs. When observing the face, don't be overly concerned with small details—look for overall signs. It is usually easy to distinguish an ill person from a healthy one. Begin to trust your native, intuitive ability and use it in choosing the type of treatment you give. Don't analyze and think too much.

Type of Treatment

Shiatsu is easy to learn. You don't need much technical

knowledge. No tools or special equipment are necessary to do a treatment. Your hands and your body are the tools that you use.

The actual techniques that we use will be much the same for each person, but it is the *manner* in which we apply the technique that is different. Chronically ill or weak people should receive less physical pressure during the treatment. Instead they should be treated with a holding technique in order to increase their energy and to regain normal balance. This soft approach, without strong gripping strength, tonifies and strengthens the body.

In contrast, stronger people, especially those who are large, overweight, and stiff, need more pressure and a vigorous treatment style. They have excessive energy which has stagnated, causing stiffness. The purpose of using pressure with them is to decrease this excessive energy and regain normal balance.

When working with the elderly, children, or pregnant women, we must look at each case, use common sense, and decide how to treat each one individually. Care and a delicate touch are generally recommended. If you are uncertain how much pressure is correct, you can safely use palm healing—a gentle, touch technique— without any worry. These three groups respond better to a softer treatment (see Palm Healing in the next chapter).

For serious illnesses, such as cancer, AIDS (acquired immune deficiency syndrome), etc., the same is true. If you are uncertain about how to treat, you can safely do a holding technique such as palm healing. These soft styles exchange energy rather than pressure. If, during the shiatsu session, you feel that one or some of the techniques are too difficult for the receiver, then use your common sense and skip that technique. If the person is weak, there is no need to do all the techniques that are described, as this may tire them.

The macrobiotic approach to shiatsu is to use the simplest techniques that we know. It is easiest to allow natural force to do the work for us. The better our technique, the less effort we have to use. Our technical form is more important than the force of physical power.

The Two Phases of Treatment

Each treatment has two parts. The first phase loosens and relaxes the receiver. This both increases circulation and softens the body. The second phase treats the whole body and specific, troubled areas, such as tightness in the neck or a poorly functioning internal organ.

The Loosening Phase

Some areas of the body easily become stiff and tight. This is a common result of overuse. If you use your right hand frequently without trying to equalize the work by using the left hand, you can develop chronic sore arm, shoulder or neck problems. Sometimes, body fluids pool in certain areas, creating swelling, congestion, and poor circulation. The loosening phase of the treatment is a good safeguard against swelling. The receiver can be in any position, but the lying down posture is most effective. This non-specific treatment normally takes between three to five minutes, but can be done in as little as one minute. It is safe and easy. You can use your hands or feet. Because of the dense nerve mass in the spine, we can stimulate the central nervous system by pressing this area (see page 77, back treatment in full shiatsu chapter). This relaxes the entire body and adjusts the functions of the internal organs. Simply press the back while leaning your body weight into it, working either up or down the spine. The amount of pressure should be governed by intuition and experience.

Whole Body Phase

The second phase of the session treats the whole body. A full body session includes the neck, shoulders, back, abdomen, arms, legs, and head. Pressing and massaging all the various body parts creates an integrated, whole feeling for the receiver. It is also the most effective way to achieve balance. If you don't have enough time to do a complete session, then you can go directly to the troubled area.

Shiatsu massage uses touch pressure to alter the condition within the body. This improves circulation of blood and lymph fluids as well as the unseen energy that moves within us. Shiatsu has several functions. The four main ones are:

1. To easily create a state of relaxation;
2. To increase circulation throughout the body, including the muscles and internal organs, and to promote flexibility of the joints;
3. To regulate proper nerve function through the central nervous system and the autonomic nervous system;
4. To strengthen the body's ability to resist disease.

A shiatsu treatment uses various types of pressure techniques. Each has its own effect. These same techniques can be used for self-shiatsu.

Touch Techniques

With barefoot shiatsu we use many types of touching techniques. They are: holding or palm healing, touching, vibrating, shaking, rubbing, kneading, tapping, "leaning into it", and bending and stretching. The energy that we use to accomplish our tasks comes from our body's center—the area located just below the navel.

Named the *hara* in Oriental medicine, this area is thought to be a principle storage place of energy as well as the physical center of the body. It is here that we have our balancing point. Before you even touch the giver, concentrate your energy in the lower abdomen and allow it to flow from there to your hands. Never just use the pressure from the fingers, hands, or feet. Rather, by leaning into the touch with an exhalation, the weight of the giver's body brings about a beneficial effect. Finger-tip pressure alone causes pain and has less benefit.

Holding - Palm Healing

This method is used when we want to transfer or stimulate energy movement in someone. In palm healing, the hand is placed on the receiver's body. The giver relaxes, breathes deep, rhythmic breaths and concentrates on sending healing energy to the receiver. The breath is quiet and the exhalation longer then the receiver's. Just hold the hand near the area of treatment. This can be done with or without actually touching. This technique is used when someone has cancer, AIDS, or skin disorders such as burns, cuts or rashes, or even stomachache. Holding can be used with anyone, especially with older people and children.

Touching

The act of touching brings a subtle response from the body. Touching brings about a sense of trust and confidence between people. When we pat someone on the back or shake hands during an introduction, we are using the touching method. When you concentrate on your palm and touch, the receiver's body becomes synchronized and balanced. Continue touching until you feel satisfied then move to the next area.

Vibrating

When doing this technique, keep your spine straight. Lightly put your hand on the receiver's skin. Your arms should be extended. Inhale and exhale with a calm, long breath. If you practice this many times with concentration, a natural vibration occurs in your hand. This vibration comes from your center. The energy transmitted from the center through the hand moves like electricity into the receiver's body. Strong concentration and practice, coordinated with breathing, is necessary to be effective. This technique is different from shaking.

Shaking

The shaking motion is used when there is a lack of vital energy within the body. This is the easiest way to loosen up any part of the body. It loosens and relaxes. The hands or feet can be used to do this simple technique.

Rubbing

Perhaps the most familiar form of touch is rubbing. When we are cold we rub the palms of our hands together. As it stimulates blood flow, rubbing is used to relieve fatigue and to improve the tone of the skin and muscles. When rubbing, place the hands flat on the body and maintain a steady pressure from the beginning to the end of the motion.

Kneading

Using the thumb and index finger together or the whole hand, knead areas such as the tendons near joints, e.g., the knee or elbow. Kneading can also be used along the back or side of the neck and along the tops of the shoulders. This squeeze motion loosens stiffness and increases circulation in the area.

Tapping

Tapping can be done with the fingers, with the palm, with the side or back of the hand, or with the fist. This light pounding should be done rhythmically. Light tapping restores vitality to tired muscles and nerves. Excessively heavy striking will tire the muscles and nerves and cause pain.

"Leaning into it"

This pressing technique is the one most frequently used in shiatsu. With the palm of the hand, the sole of the foot, or the thumbs and fingers, the whole body leans into each movement. Each press is done with coordinated exhalations of both the giver and receiver. This makes the receiver's muscles relax and the giver can get in more deeply with greater effect. Pressure comes from the center of the body not just the fingertips or feet.

Bending and Stretching

These techniques are used to increase movement and flexibility and also to relax the muscles and tendons of the joints. Upon awakening in the morning we all stretch; it is a natural process. This promotes circulation to all parts of the body. It also stimulates the body's energy channels and the acupoints simultaneously.

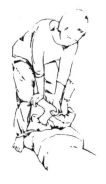
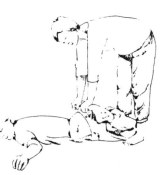

Complete Shiatsu Treatment

The full shiatsu session which follows is described in a step-by-step manner. Each step has either a photograph or illustration and a written explanation. This simple approach gives you the ability to practice directly . Look carefully at the photographs for fine points of body posture for both the giver and receiver. Photos and drawings make good, long-lasting impressions on the mind.

The written portion has key words at each step of the treatment. After you have given several treatments, a glance at the photograph and the beginning words of each step should remind you of what to do next. Eventually, the book will become unnecessary except for review and reminders. After giving several sessions, your intuition will develop.

Repetition and practice promote this development. Never miss an opportunity to help someone with shiatsu; you will both benefit.

As mentioned earlier, it is helpful to coordinate your breath during treatment. This means that both the giver and the receiver are to breathe in and out together. This strengthens the shiatsu press which takes place during the out breath. The giver tells the receiver when to breathe during this technique. So say "breathe in...." This lets the receiver know when you want him or her to follow a special breath.

Full Body Treatment

Seated Postion for Neck and Shoulders

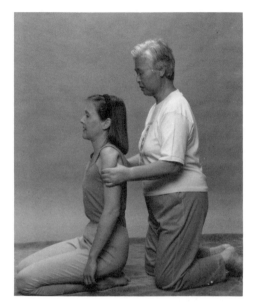

1. Have the receiver assume a seated position, either on the floor or in a chair. From behind, take hold of the arms just below the shoulders and lift up and down, loosening the shoulders. This also relaxes the nerves.

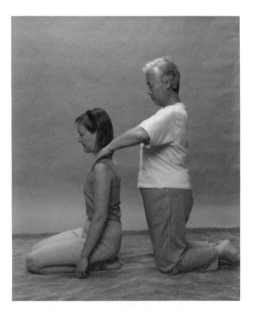

2. Knead the shoulders, with the thumbs pressing the large muscles across the top of the back. Move from the inside toward the outside. This quickly softens stiff shoulders.

3. Pound the shoulders with the sides of the hands or fists, releasing tension (illustrations 3a and 3b).

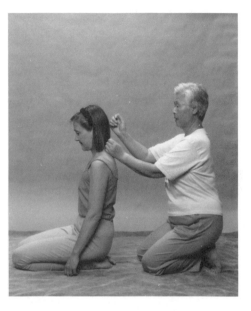

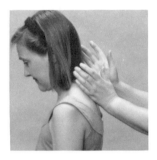

4. Press the large muscles on the side of the neck with the thumb. Press from beneath the ear to the shoulder. One hand holds the forehead slightly pushing the head backwards, while the other hand presses the neck. Do both sides of the neck by moving to the other side of the body and use the other hand. This loosens up the neck.

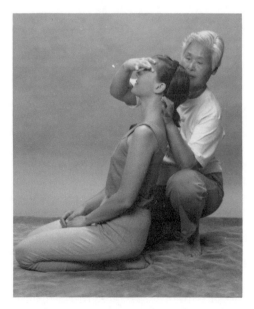

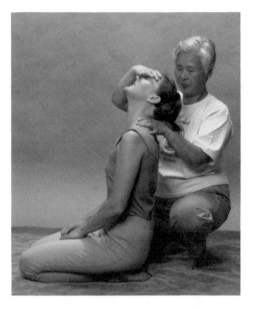

5. Rotate head by placing one hand on the forehead and the other hand on the back of the neck. Rotate in each direction three times. This releases head tension and increases neck flexibility.

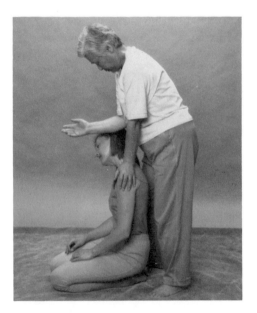

6. Stretch the neck and shoulder by placing the palm of the hand flat on the shoulder edge, and the side of the forearm against the side of the head. Inhale together and on the exhale, stretch the head away from the shoulder. Repeat on other side. Effective to loosen tight neck and shoulders.

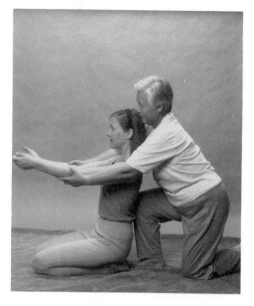

7. From behind, support receiver with one knee, as you take hold of the forearm near the elbow. Breathe in and, on the exhalation, pull the elbows back as the receiver brings the head back. This releases upper body tension which loosens up back, chest, shoulders, and neck.

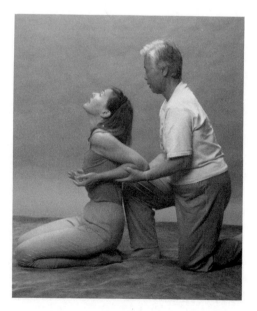

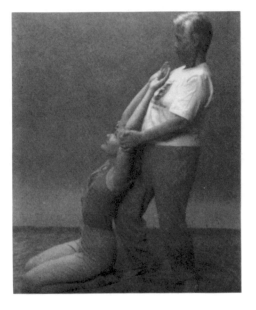

8. Standing from behind, reach over and hold the receiver's wrist. Breathe in together and, on an exhalation, lean back stretching the arms overhead. This loosens and stretches arms and chest.

Lying Down Position for Back and Lower Part of Body

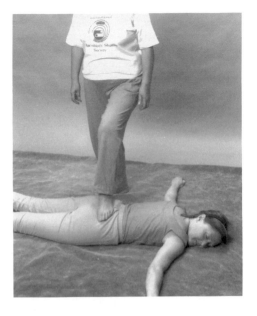

Have the receiver lie face down, with toes turned in and arms straight out at a ninety degree angle to the rest of the body.

9. Stand to the side at the waist, and roll the pelvis with the foot. This will loosen and relax the whole body quickly.

10. Standing between the receiver's legs, facing outward, walk on the bottoms of both feet at the same time, walking from arch to heel several times. Do not walk on the toes. Shift your weight from one side to the other. Your toes are on the floor; your heels do the pressing. This brings blood down from the upper body.

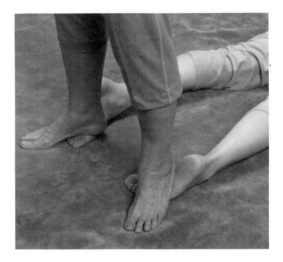

11.Press out the heel with your foot. With your right foot press down and outward lightly, to stretch out the ankle. Repeat on other side.

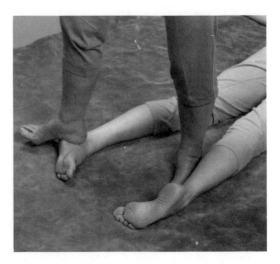

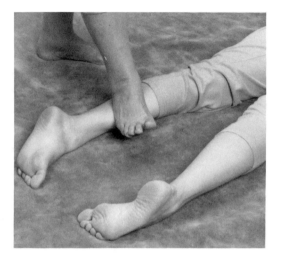

12. Walk up the calf with foot. Stand to the left side of receiver. With your right foot press down on the Achilles tendon. Then, starting close to the heel, press the leg and calf muscles with the heel of your foot up to just below the knee. Never press on the knee! This relaxes and loosens up legs.

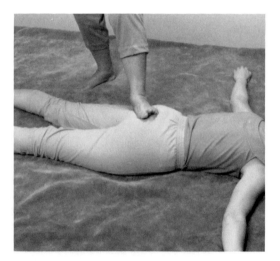

13. Change feet and press buttock with left foot. Then press the left thigh down to the knee. Repeat. Effective for relieving nervous tension.

Go to the receiver's right side and repeat same procedure. Press the Achilles tendon, then walk up the lower leg to the knee. Press the buttock and walk down the thigh to the knee (see numbers 9-13).

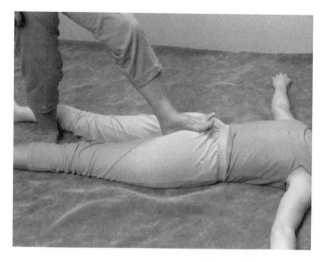

14. Stand between the receiver's legs, facing toward the head. Place your heel on the tailbone (coccyx) and quickly and gently press this area. Stimulation here relaxes nerve centers in the body. Also press around the inner thighs of both legs.

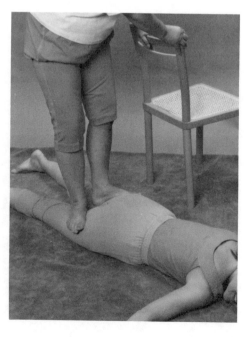

15a. Walk on upper thigh while gripping a chair to support your weight. Shift your weight from side to side as you walk down the legs. Good for loosening up leg muscles.

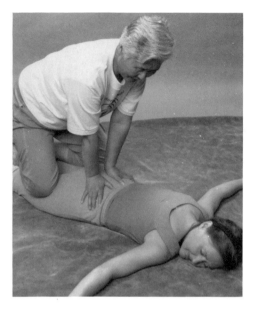

15b. As an alternative to using a chair you can use your knees to press the thighs. Support yourself with hands on receiver's hips. Press your knees on the thighs. Shift your weight from side to side.

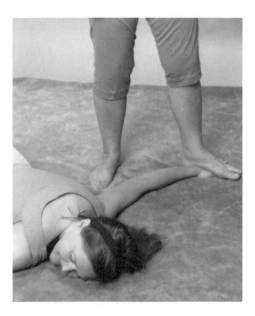

16. Stand behind the receiver's left arm. Press the hand with your foot. This relaxes hand, brain, and strengthens heart.

17. With left foot, press arm from below shoulder to wrist. Avoid the elbow! Good for bursitis and tennis elbow. Change to right side. Repeat. Press hand, then, press from below shoulder down to wrist.

Upper Part of Body

18. Standing over the receiver, with one foot on each side of the body, place the heels of your hands together at your wrist on the spine near the top of the back. Your fingers are out-stretched and perpendicular to the spine. Lean your body weight onto the receiver on an exhalation. Move your hands down from the shoulder blade region to the waist, one breath at a time. This loosens up the back.

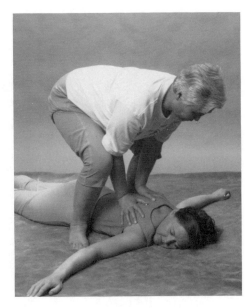

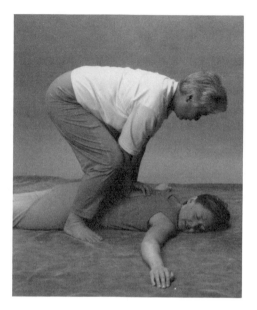

19. Press the back down the center of the spine with one palm on top of the other. Lean your body weight on the back, pressing on an exhalation. OR you can choose to:

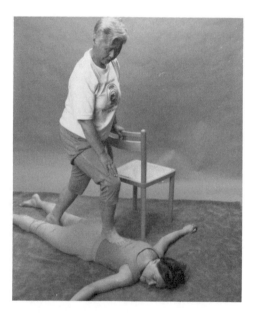

20. Stand to the side of receiver. With the ball of the foot, press down the spine, leaning into it. Move from between the shoulder blades to the waist. OR as an alternative you can:

21. Use a chair for balance, step up on the buttocks near the hip with most of the weight. With one foot near the hip, use the other foot to press gently, moving down from between the shoulder blades to the waist. Press and hold each position for 1-2 seconds. All three methods loosen up the back and can correct spinal alignment.

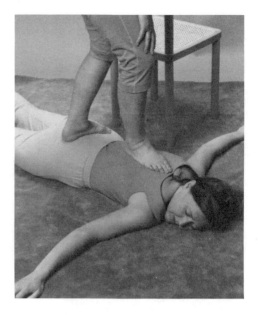

22. Standing on the receiver, using a chair for balance, allow your toes to press into the lower back just above the hipbone. Gently rock and loosen this area. Good for stiff hip and relaxing the lower back. Also effects abdominal and menstrual cramps.

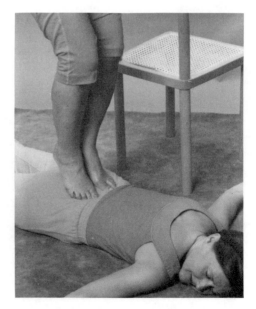

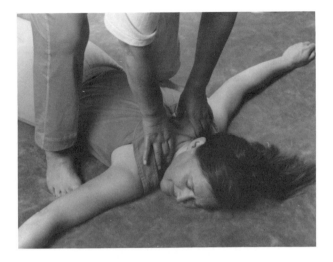

23. Standing with one foot on each side of the receiver, bend over and knead the shoulders.

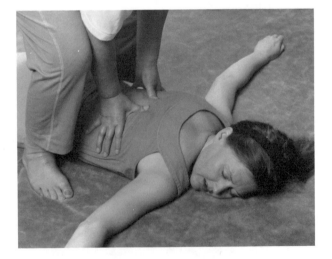

24. Use the thumbs to press the acupuncture energy lines on the back. Beginning near the large bone at the shoulder level in the center of the back, place the thumbs 1 1/2 inches from the spine. Breathe in together and on an exhalation press straight down, leaning your body weight into it. Hold each point for 3-5 seconds. Continue down the back at each vertebra to the tailbone. Carefully observe body posture. Press the second line, three inches away from the spine as before. Repeat both lines.

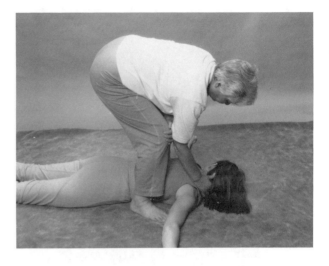

25. Press temples of the head and the arch around the ears with the thumb. Hold each point for several seconds. Turn head and do other side. Good for headaches and ear and hearing troubles.

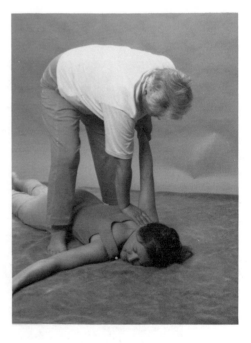

26. Place your right hand at the receiver's left shoulder. With the left hand take the wrist and lift it, stretching the arm. Rotate it several times in both directions.

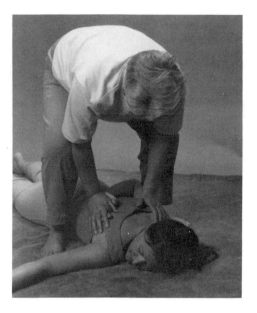

27. Bend the arm at the elbow and place the hand as far up on the back as is comfortable.

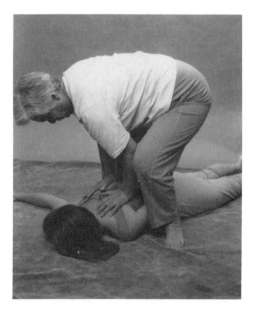

28a. Hold the receiver's left hand with your right hand. Place your left hand on the shoulder blade. Lean your body weight here. Press in and down toward the center, loosening the shoulder blade.

28b. Press with your thumb along the contour of the shoulder blade.

Treatment numbers 26-29 are very effective for stiff shoulder and shoulder joint problems.

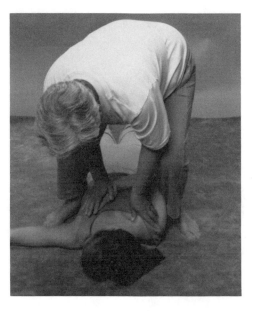

29. Adjust the shoulder by pushing the arm upward toward the back of the neck quickly and release.

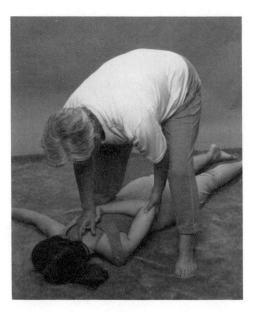

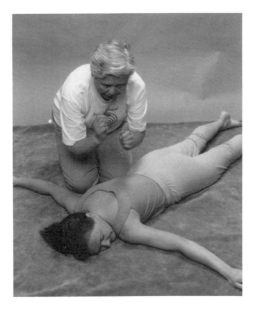

Change arms and repeat. Bend the arm at the elbow, lean your body weight on the shoulder blade, press with the thumb around the shoulder blade and adjust the arm stretch. (See numbers 26-29)

30 a. Go to the side of receiver and gently pound the back with lightly closed fists.

30 b. You can also pound with your palms together, lightly striking the back with the back of the hands. This is an easy technique to relax the back. It also improves circulation.

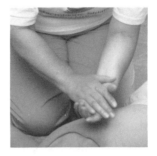

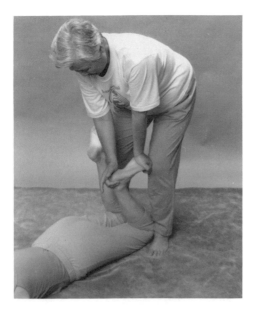

31. Go to the feet of the receiver and bend the leg at the knee. With one foot up in the air at a time, grab and bend the toes toward the floor. This will stretch the Achilles tendon and ankle.

32. With the receiver's knees bent, grip the toes of each foot and lean your body weight on the legs, bending them onto the buttocks.

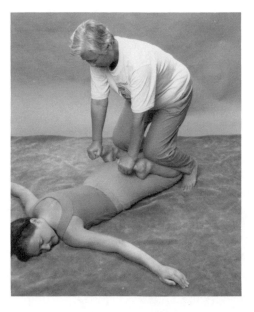

33. Cross the ankles and push the legs onto the buttocks again. Reverse the ankles and repeat the downward stretch.

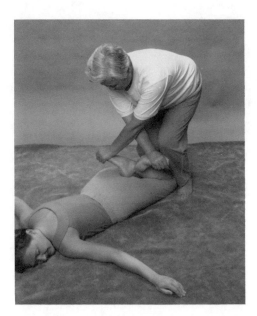

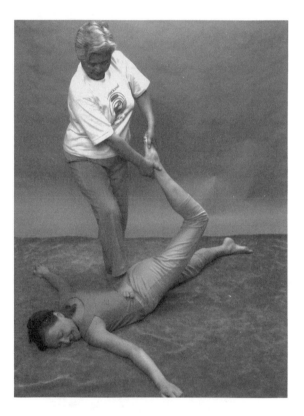

34. Straighten the legs. Hold the left ankle. Place your right foot on top of the pelvic bone. Pull upward, diagonally, stretching the leg. Return the leg to its resting position. Repeat this from the other side with the other leg. Carefully observe photograph for correct body posture. You can move your support foot on the back. Move from pelvic area upward. This stretches the whole body.

Front Side and the Lower Part of the Body

35. Have receiver turn over onto the back. Stand at the feet of the receiver. Bend both knees and push down toward the chest on an exhalation. This stretches the lower back and loosens and increases flexibility in the hips.

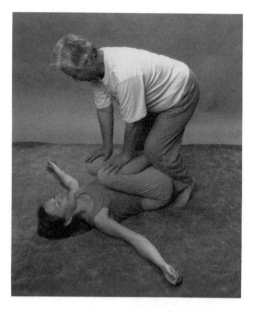

36. Hold same position and rotate the knees in both clockwise (a.) and counterclockwise (b.) directions.

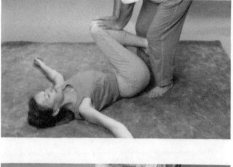

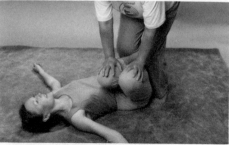

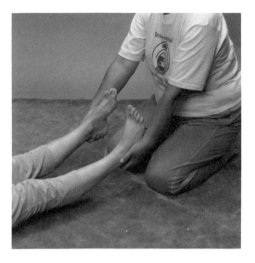

37. Sit at the receiver's feet. Hold both legs at the ankles and lift them off the floor. Sway back and forth, open the legs and drop the feet.

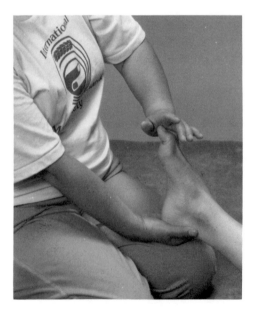

38. Pick up the right foot. Hold it with the right hand. With your left hand brush the toes.

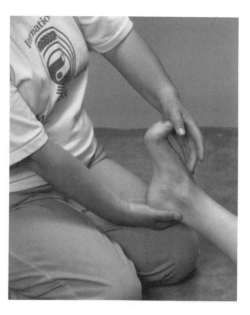

39a. Bend the toes in one direction.

39b. Bend them in the opposite direction.

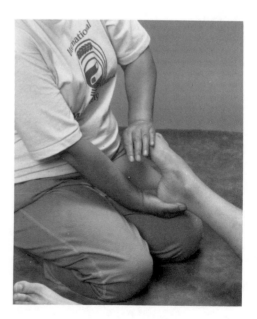

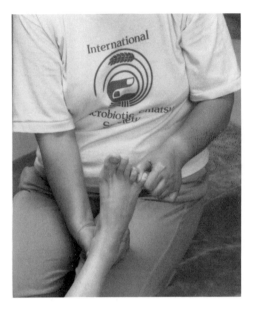

40. Manipulate each toe by pressing from top and bottom and side to side. This stimulates all internal organs.

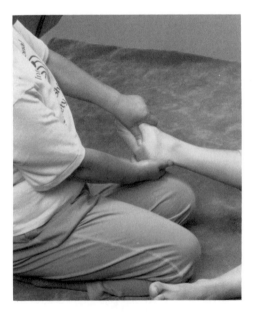

41. Turn the foot to the side and press the sole. You can also pound the sole of the foot. This has good effect on mental fatigue as it stimulates vital organs.

42. Rotate the ankle in each direction.

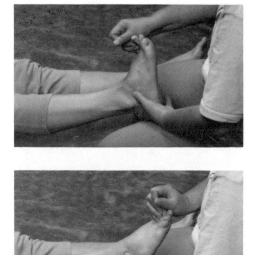

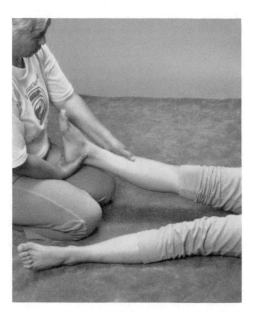

43. Massage the top of the leg on the shinbone from inside the ankle to below the knee. Press with both thumb on top and index finger on bottom making small circles.

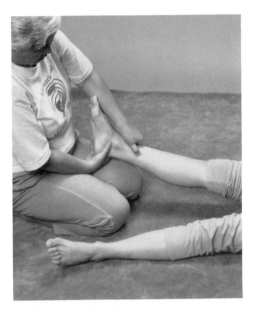

44. Press up under the shinbone on inside of the leg from the ankle to below the knee.

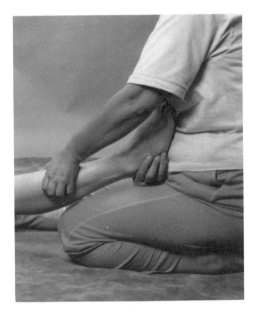

45. Wrap four fingers of your left hand around the outside of the middle leg. Press from ankle to below the knee.

46. Change hands. From the inside, squeeze the calf and Achilles tendon.

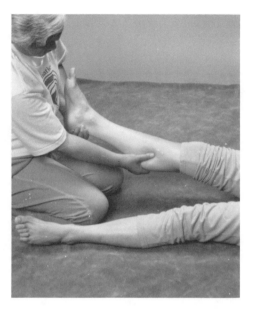

47. Press with the thumb on the outside of the shinbone from below the knee to the ankle.

Pick up other foot and repeat from beginning (numbers 37-47).

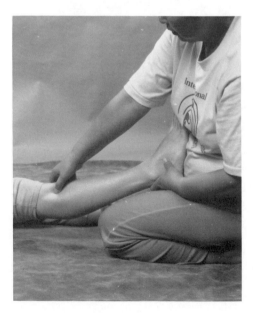

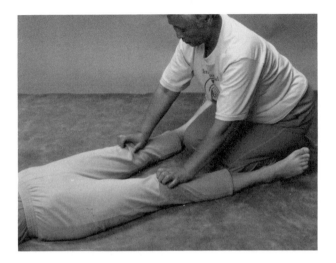

48. Move up between the receiver's legs. Place palm over the knee caps and press back and forth. Good for any knee trouble.

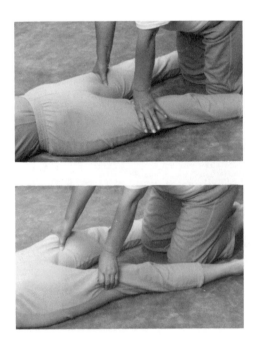

49. Squeeze the thighs from above the knee to the pelvis. With the thumb and index finger, squeeze while body weight is leaning onto the thighs. Especially in the groin area, use thumbs to press lymph nodes. This softens the muscles by increasing circulation and distributes energy throughout the body.

50. Lightly bend knee, holding toe and ankle. Quickly pull and adjust ankle.

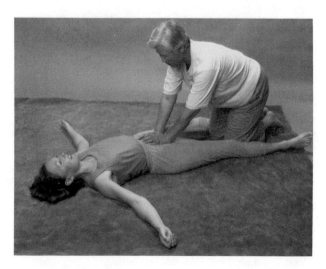

51. Press abdomen by placing one palm down with the other on top just above the pubic bone. Coordinate the breath and on an exhalation press down. Repeat up to three times. This stimulates and strengthens the internal organs.

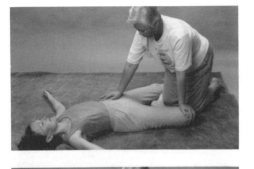

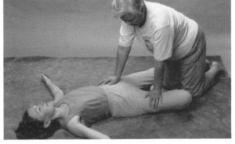

52a. Rotate knee outward, allowing it to go to the floor.

52b. Press with the palm of the hand moving up toward the hip,

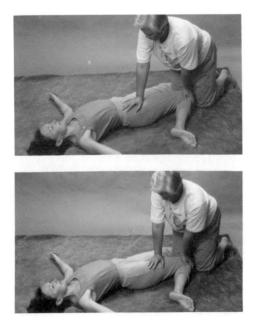

53a. Rotate knee inward, allowing it to go to the floor.

53b. Press with the palm of the hand moving downward from the hip toward the knee.

Numbers 52 and 53 loosen up hips and are good for joints.

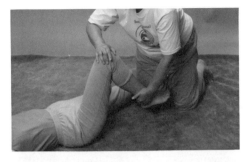

54. Hold ankle and knee. Pull out ankle and stretch knee.

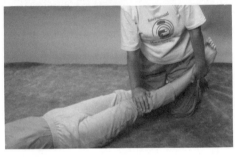

Upper Part of Body

55. With thumbs on top and fingers beneath on the palm, squeeze and bend the hand, relaxing it.

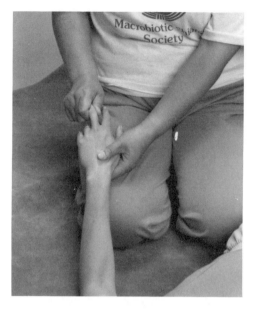

56. Manipulate each finger individually. Start with the small finger. Press top and bottom at the same time. Effects internal organs.

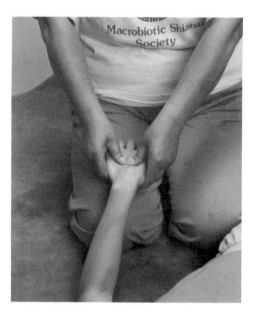

57. With thumb, press the top of the hand from the wrist toward each finger. Treating the hand is very effective in combating fatigue.

58. Turn palm up. Place the little finger of your outside hand between the receiver's little and ring fingers. Place the little finger of your other hand between the receiver's index finger and thumb. Spread and stretch the palm.

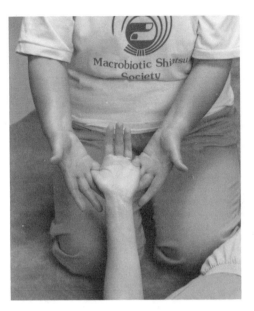

59. Press this palm area with both your thumbs. Treating the center of the palm is especially good for the heart.

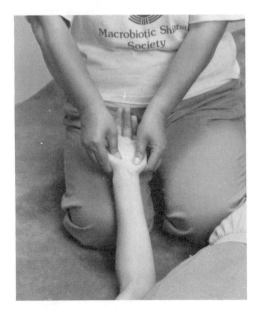

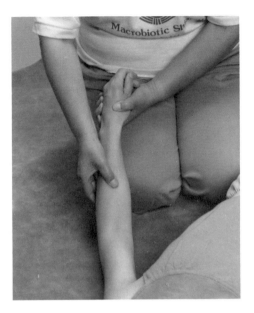

60. Hold the receiver's left hand. Press simultaneously top and bottom with your thumb and index finger directly on top of the wrist-bone and the back of the arm. Manipulate from the wrist up to the elbow. Repeat several times.

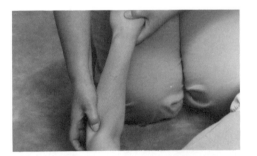

61. Press on a diagonal from the inside wrist toward the outside elbow on top of the forearm. Repeat several times.

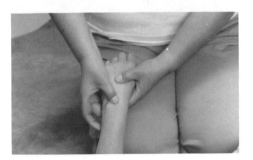

62. Turn the palm up and press directly up the middle of the arm, both top and bottom, to the elbow.

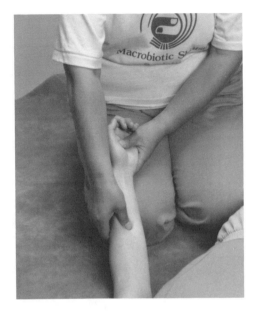

63. Press, squeeze, and massage the upper arm. Beginning at the top of the shoulder, press until you reach the elbow. Hold each point for 1-3 seconds.

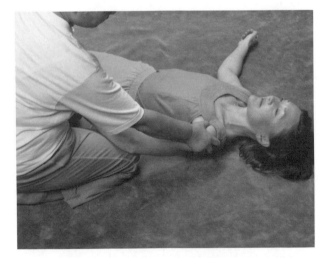

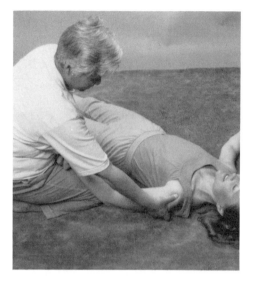

64a. Begin at the shoulder again, this time beginning slightly higher near the top of the shoulder.

64b. Press down to the elbow moving along the outside of the upper arm.
Repeat several times.

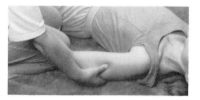

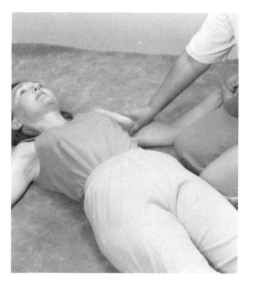

65. Press in the underarm from inside the shoulder down to the elbow. Repeat several times.

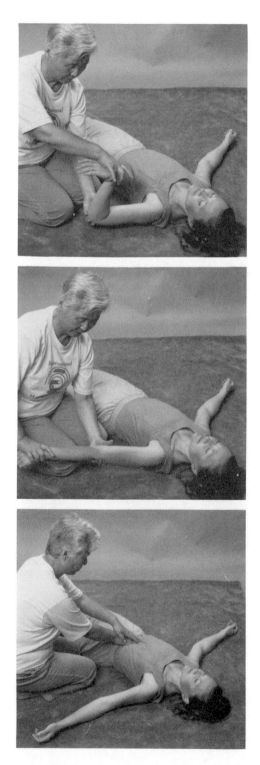

66a. Bend elbow and hold wrist as seen in photograph.

66b. Adjust the arm by pulling the wrist outward parallel with the floor. Release the arm.

Face the receiver's trunk area directly so that you can work on the abdomen.

67. With your outstretched fingers, probe the abdomen to get a general idea of its condition. Be attentive to hard, soft, hot, or cold areas.

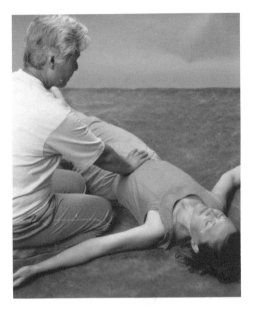

68. With the heel of your right hand placed directly on the abdomen, massage in a clockwise direction. Massage within the area made by the ribs and hip bones. This relaxes abdominal muscles, increases circulation and assimilation, and helps constipation.

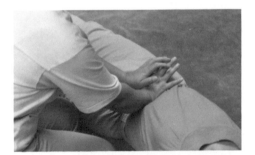

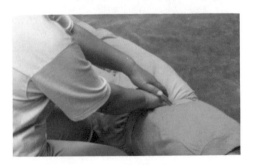

69. Knead the intestines as you lean your weight into the receiver's navel area. Gently, but deeply, knead as you would bread dough. The hands remain in one place. Push with the heel of your hand and pull with the finger-tips. This strongly stimulates internal organs.

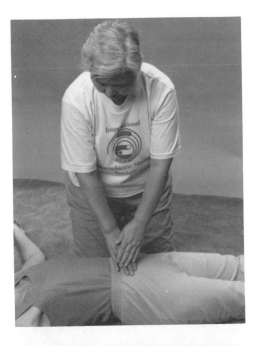

70. Place your palms on the abdomen. Coordinate your breathing with the receiver's breathing. On exhaling, press down gently until you feel resistance. Hold for 1-3 seconds. On inhaling, lift the palms off. Repeat up to ten times. This increases overall energy and balances the body. It also brings deep relaxation.

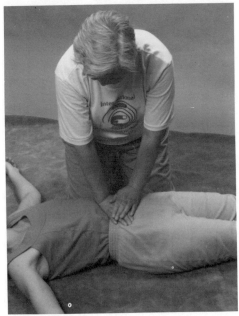

Move to the receiver's right side. Kneel between the body and the outstretched arm. Massage the left hand as you did the other hand (number 55).

Massage the lower and upper arms as you did on the other side (numbers 56-65). Adjust the arm by bending it and pulling the wrist in an outward direction (Number 66) Put arm down on the floor.

Move to Behind the Receiver's Head.

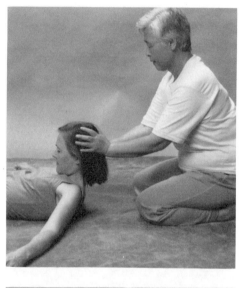

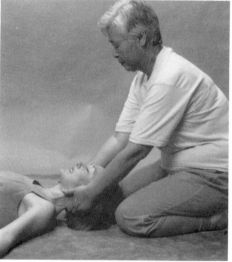

71. Pick up the head with both hands and stretch the neck by moving the head toward the chest. Try to touch the chin to the chest.

72. Place hands under the neck and pull the head toward yourself, stretching the neck and body.

73. While holding the head, rotate it in a figure eight, moving the chin from side to side (no photograph).

74a. Place the head on the floor and, with the bottom of your fist, gently and rhythmically pound the sides and top of the head.

74b. You can tap with the side of your open hand. You can also press the top of the head with the thumbs. These are good for mental fatigue. They also affect sinus congestion and internal organs.

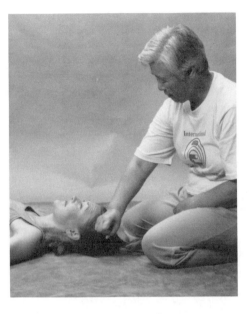

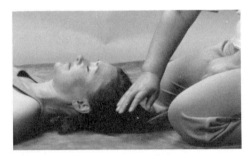

Face and Head

Use thumb and finger pressure to stimulate the face. Hold each point for 3-5 seconds.

75. Start with the thumbs on the inside corner of the eyebrow. Press along the eyebrows and onto the forehead.

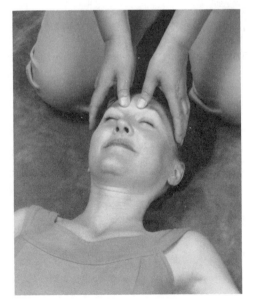

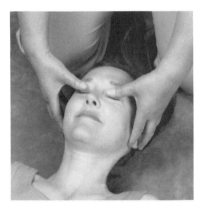

76. Gently press with the thumbs over the eyeball and around the eyes.

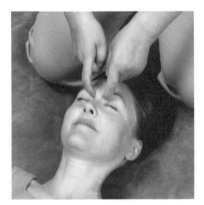

77. Press with the index fingers in the inside corner of the eye. If you feel tightness, loosen it.

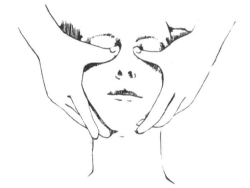

78. Press under the eye rim. This stimulates tear ducts and sinus regions.

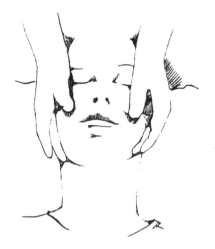

79. Press around the cheek-bone, hold each point for 2-5 seconds. This helps sinus congestion.

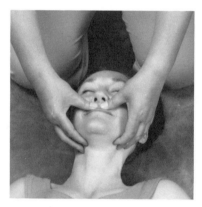

80. Press the groove under the nose. This balances the nervous system.

81. With the thumbs, press around the mouth. Good for digestive system and toothache.

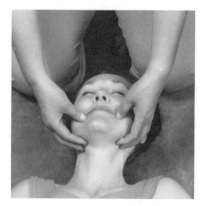

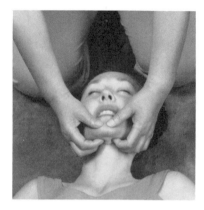

82. With the thumbs on the topside and the fingers wrapped under, press the chin and jaw.

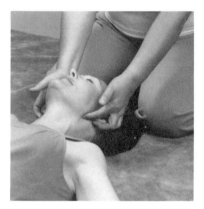

83. With index fingertips, press the indentation in back of the ear at the lower border. This stimulates the lymph nodes and alleviates toothache.

84. Press, massage and pull the ears. Effects the whole body. It is especially good for ear trouble.

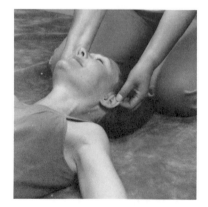

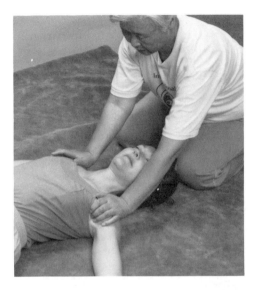

85. Place your hands on the receiver's shoulders and push them toward the feet. This shaking and pushing will loosen the neck and shoulders.

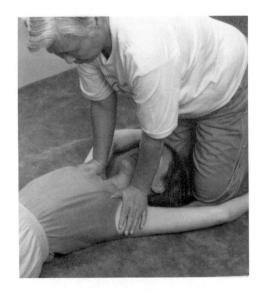

86. Bring the arms over the head. Press the armpit and lymph nodes. This also loosens shoulder joints.

87. Holding the arms at the wrist, have the receiver breathe in. On an exhalation, you pull the arms outstretched, while the receiver pushes the heels out. The toes are pointed toward the body. This is a very good overall body stretch.

End of Treatment

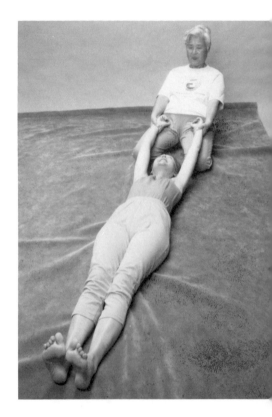

Moxibustion

The healing effect of heat has been known to mankind since our primitive beginnings. When ancient man discovered fire to cook his food, many more items, especially tough, fibrous root vegetables, could be included in the diet, with added vitamins, minerals, and calories.

But the use of fire has developed beyond warming ourselves and cooking our food. According to Chinese historians, a remedy for abdominal symptoms was discovered accidentally; in primitive times people noticed that when they warmed themselves by the fire, they experienced relief from abdominal pains, distention and fullness. In this way moxibustion, the application of heat to a specific area of the body for the purpose of treating illness, evolved. It is still an important part of Chinese medicine along with herbs, diet, exercise, massage, and acupuncture. In fact the Chinese word that is translated as acupuncture, *Zhen Jiu,* actually means needle (*zhen*) and moxibustion (*jiu*).

Mugwort (artemisia vulgaris) is the plant commonly used for this burning technique. The sun-dried leaves are powdered to a fluffy or wooly consistency and applied to the acupuncture points as well as other areas of the body. Moxibustion can be used either directly on the skin or, more commonly, indirectly with some material first placed on the skin directly under the burning moxa. Ginger, garlic, and sea salt have all been used for various effects. The method which is easiest to use, and the one that we recommend for home use, is the cigar method. The moxa is rolled like a large cigar, lit, and held over the area where treatment is desired.

Moxibustion heat warms the vital energy (*ki* or *qi*) and blood in the acupuncture channels. It is especially good for chronic weak conditions. It improves the circulation of both blood and vital energy. In practice, it is used for asthma, diarrhea, arthritis, rheumatic pain, vomiting, abdominal pain, and women's problems (such as painful menstruation). After shiatsu treatment some specific areas of the body may need more attention. Moxibustion is useful at that time.

How to Use Moxibustion

Moxa rolls are the most convenient way to apply moxibustion. The receiver can be treated in any position which is comfortable. The end of the moxa roll is ignited to give an even, red glow. It may be necessary to peel off some of the outer paper on the moxa roll, which allows it to burn more strongly. After the end is lit, the roll can be held near the acupoint or area that you wish to treat. Warm the area with either a circular movement or bird-pecking movement until the spot is sufficiently warmed. For the bird-pecking movement, bring the roll slowly near and then away from the skin repeatedly so that the receiver feels a pleasant warmth. The roll will come to within one inch of the skin surface. Never leave it so close to the skin and for so long that the receiver complains of too much heat pain. Ask the receiver to tell you when it is hot. The treatment is very warming and comfortable. It should be continued for about five to ten minutes in each area.

Care must be taken throughout the session not to burn the receiver nor to allow the ash to fall on the receiver. An ashtray should be near you so that you can knock off the ash occasionally. Moxa rolls may be snuffed out in a candlestick holder or by making a cap of aluminum foil. Do not put the roll in water. They should be stored in a dry place.

If moxa rolls can not be obtained in your area, you can use cigarettes for the same purpose. However, moxa is far superior. Check oriental herb shops, acupuncture supply companies, and East-West Centers for moxa sales.

Do not use moxibustion for the following conditions:

1. Pregnant Women. Do not use moxa on the abdomen and back areas.   However, it may be used safely on the arms and legs.

2. On the Face. Don't use moxa on the face, especially around the eyes.

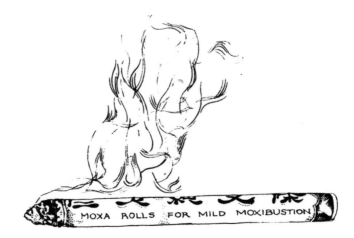

MOXA ROLLS FOR MILD MOXIBUSTION

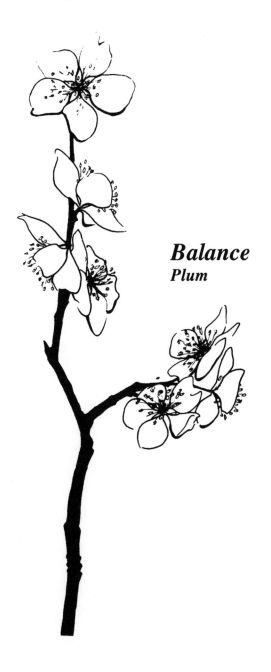

Balance
Plum

Treating Common Problems

Many people from time to time suffer from a variety of common complaints. These typical problems, found within the family, are covered in this section.

The source of most of our imbalance is simply blockage. It can be a blockage of a physical or energetic nature. Mucous, fat, or poor energy circulation contribute to this stagnation. Blockage within and around the organs, as well as within the muscles and nervous and circulatory systems, interferes with the good functioning of the body and mind. The circulation of energy must go well for an organ to function well, and therefore for balance to be maintained. Disruption in the flow of energy lessens vitality. When this happens, you don't feel well.

Energy comes from heaven and earth. Without energy (*Ki* or *Qi*), nothing would exist. Specifically, energy comes from genetic inheritance, the food that we eat, the air that we breath, and the movement activities that we do. Your perception of an increase or decrease in energy is a notation of normal body adjustment that continually goes on. Through our daily activities we create energy. It flows throughout the body in specific pathways or channels. This ancient knowledge of energy circulation has been known and passed down for thousands of years. We are not only bones, muscles, nor nerves. We are the total of these sources of energy. As blockage interrupts the flow of energy, biological function is slowed down and problems arise.

It is important to understand this simple and basic approach of traditional medicine. With this understanding it is clear that if the flow of energy can be changed, then the physical, mental, or emotional trouble can be changed. In other words, as you remove the obstruction to normal energy flow your health improves. For example, if your car is not working well and you check and discover that the oil and air filters are dirty, you change them, thereby improving the performance of the car. By simply removing the obstructions the automobile functions better.

We are not only using western medicine or oriental medicine. We are combining the two to synthesize a more total approach. Our aim is to help understand our human place within nature.

Each condition listed in this chapter has suggestions for treatment including shiatsu, diet, exercise, moxibustion, special food preparations, and external treatments. If when viewing a problem we can see the existing stagnation of energy, then the appropriateness of these simple solutions is clear.

Some conditions demand a long-term commitment to achieve results. The effects of frequent shiatsu are enhanced by exercise and dietary adjustments. The receiver must be encouraged towards self-healing by adding as many natural methods prescribed for a given condition as possible. In this way, improvement is faster and more certain. A helpful word of encouragement from you to the receiver will give him or her confidence in the treatment and the healing process.

The Internal Organs

According to traditional Chinese medicine, the internal organs are connected to one another, as well as to the surface of the body, by a system of channels through which vital energy flows. The channels form a network that helps to regulate the function of the whole body. Each organ is supplied with energy by its own channel. Additional smaller channels connect the different organs. Because of the direct connection between two organs, they can affect each other's function. There is a close relationship between them. Because of this relationship they are considered paired organs.

Together with the ten organs there are two functions that are recognized in traditional Chinese medicine. These two functions also have channels for energy circulation. The Heart Governor controls blood circulation and relates to physical and emotional aspects of the heart. The Triple Heater coordinates all body functions. Both of these functions are extremely important in the well-being of the individual.

The following chart shows the paired organs—e.g., Lung and Large Intestine— and the flow of energy throughout the body in a continuous cycle. Troubles that affect the intestine will interfere with the function of the lung and vice versa. This relationship is true for all the paired organs. In other words, kidney trouble can show symptoms in the bladder; heart trouble can affect the small intestine and digestion; nervous stomach can affect the function of the pancreas, and so forth. (See Chart on following page.)

Simplifed Functions of the Internal Organs
and
Energy Flow

Lung [1]—internalizes *Ki* and air → **Large Intestine**[2]— absorbs
and removes waste   glucose, salt, and liquid,
                                         removes waste, aids lung

Stomach [2]—receives and digests → **Pancreas/Spleen** [1]—makes
food   hormones and digestive liquid

Heart [1]—circulates blood,   → **Small Intestine** [2]—absorbs nutri-
maintains emotional stability   ents from food, creates blood with
                                            the bone marrow

Urinary Bladder [2]—stores and → **Kidney** [1]—filters and cleans the
passes liquid waste   blood

Heart Governor [1]—governs   → **Triple Heater** [2]—regulates circu-
circulation and relates to   lation and coordinates all body
physical and emotional aspects   functions
of the heart

Gall Bladder [2]—stores bile, a   → **Liver** [1]—cleans, stores and
digestive enzyme of fat   makes blood

---

[1] Solid Organs   [2] Hollow Organs

Macrobiotic medicine designates the solid organs as *Yang* organs and the hollow organs as *Yin* organs. Traditional Chinese Medicine designates the solid organs as *Yin* organs and the hollow organs as *Yang* organs. While apparently contradictory the designations work well within the context of their use. The Chinese medical view is based on energy, while Macrobiotics emphasizes a more material approach.

Lung

chest pain
asthma
bronchitis
emphysema

The lungs are the principal organs of respiration. They fill the chest cavity, lying one on each side separated in the middle by the heart. The lungs are cone-shaped organs which have their base resting on the floor of the thoracic cavity—diaphragm. The inside of the lungs are lined with tiny air sacs called alveoli, each of which consists of a single layer of cells. It is here that the blood comes into almost direct contact with the air and an interchange of gases takes place. Oxygen from the air we breath attaches to the iron in the red blood cell in the alveoli, while, at the same time, the blood cell is getting rid of its waste material, carbon dioxide. A mucous membrane lines the bronchial tubes (air passages) and the lungs. It is covered with hair-like cells that help keep the passages clean.

When various outside substances, such as viruses, molds, bacteria, yeasts, dust, and pollen or factors taken in through food and drink, such as fatty dairy products, sugars, fruit juices, and chocolate, make contact with the mucous membrane, they can stimulate the production of excessive amounts of mucus. Excessive mucus swells the breathing passages and clogs the alveoli, interfering with the smooth exchange of gases in the normal breathing cycle. At the same time, while breathing ability is decreased because of congestion, the mucus also serves as a breeding ground for viruses and other infectious material. As this continues, breathing becomes more and more difficult, and the body begins to rid itself of the accumulated matter through coughing and sneezing. The cough or the sneeze is the first attempt by the body to heal itself by expelling the toxin filled mucus.

The aim of treatment is to encourage this natural healing process. Cleansing the lungs is accomplished by cleaning up the diet. Both the lungs and the intestines are lined with mucous membranes; the decrease of mucus production in the intestines will decrease production in the lungs. Shiatsu and ginger compresses also help speed recovery.

Diet

The avoidance of all artificially-produced and chemicalized foods such as ice cream, soft drinks, frozen fruit juice, sugar, and greasy, fried foods is necessary when problems like asthma, bronchitis, and emphysema are present. Instead the diet should include well prepared whole grains and fresh cooked vegetables. Additionally, miso soup with seaweed should be eaten daily. After some time of eating the macrobiotic way, your breathing will be much freer and easier as excess mucus will not be produced. Speciality items such as salted plums (*umeboshi*) can be taken, one per day, and sesame salt (approximately 14-20 parts sesame seed mixed with 1 part good quality seasalt) can be used as a condiment on whole grains and vegetables. These will help to clean the blood and contract swollen bronchi, thereby opening the breathing passages.

Shiatsu

Specific areas for shiatsu include the neck, shoulders, between the shoulder blades, and the front part of the chest. Doing the seated part of the full treatment will stimulate these areas adequately. Include shiatsu of the hands and arms, as the lung channel which travels on these body parts will affect the function of the lungs.

Standing behind the receiver, place one hand on the forehead and the thumb of the other hand on the medulla oblongata point in the center of the back of the neck. Have the receiver breathe in and, on an exhalation, gently roll the head back onto the thumb. Repeat this 5-7 times. Massage the muscles on both sides of the neck. Hold each point for several seconds and repeat 3 times.

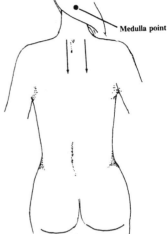

Place the thumbs near the center of the spine with the rest of the fingers resting on the shoulders. Firmly press the acupoints located between the shoulder blades. The area from the shoulder level down to the bottom of the shoulder blade refers to the lungs and heart.

Have the receiver lie on the back. Press down the center of the chest on the sternum (breast bone) using the thumb. Use the other four fingers and gently massage the chest muscles. The area in front of the shoulder specifically energizes the lungs. Press here with the thumb, holding the acupoints around the outline of the shoulder for 3-5 seconds.

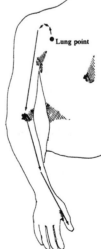

Ginger Compress

Compresses applied directly to either the front of the body on the chest, or the back on the shoulder blade area, will affect the lungs. Replace compress when it cools down, about every 30 seconds. Repeat this until lung area becomes red, about 15-20 minutes.

inflamed breast (mastitis)

Inflamed breast can occur after childbirth in breast feeding women, especially with the first child. An accumulation of mother's milk blocks the flow out of the breast. This causes the nipple to crack and become infected. An abscess can result. The skin in the area becomes red and the lymph nodes in the arm pit on the same side as the affected breast swell greatly. Some women have chills and fever.

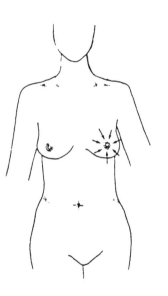

Shiatsu

Have the receiver lie on the back. The giver can apply sesame oil to the breast. Gently massage with the thumb around the lump in the breast. Then, holding the breast with the fingers of both hands, use the two thumbs in alternation to rub down along the swollen lump from the top of the lump down to the nipple. Fluid will begin to come out. Then hold the breast firmly with one hand and with the other thumb and forefingers squeeze down along the swollen mass toward the nipple. The pressure should be tolerable for the woman.

Ginger Compress

A compress can be placed directly on the affected breast to open the blocked pores.

Large Intestine

---

gas (flatulence)

colitis

constipation

hernia

diarrhea

hemorrhoids (piles)

The digestive system receives and prepares food for assimilation by the body. There are many body parts that are involved in this process. The last organ of the alimentary canal is the large intestine. The large intestine, which is about five feet long, connects with the small intestine. When food enters the stomach, the intestine is stimulated to contract and expand, which causes a defecation reflex. This stimulates the bowels. The last five inches of the large intestine make up the rectum.

The large intestine does not take part in the digestion or absorption of food. By the time that material has reached the beginning of the intestine, all the nutrients have been absorbed, and the contents are liquid. In passing through the intestine, the contents become more solid as water is absorbed. It takes about 16-24 hours for the contents to pass through the large intestine and reach the rectum.

The functions of the large intestine are to absorb water, salt, and glucose (a simple sugar) back into the body. It also prepares cellulose, which is present in grains, vegetables, and fruits, as well as any undigested protein, to be passed out of the body.

Gas may be caused by bacterial fermentation of food. Sometimes cellulose in vegetables is broken down in the intestines to produce methane and hydrogen gases. Other foul smelling gas odors, such as the rotten egg smell, comes from sulfurated hydrogen and carbon disulfate found in eggs, peas, and beans. In order to lessen intestinal gas several things are necessary. First, the intestines and the digestive system must become stronger. Secondly, the cooking preparation of both high cellulose vegetables, such as whole grains and beans, must be done correctly. Proper cooking of these foods allows the gases to be changed before you eat them. Thorough chewing is the last step in minimizing gas production inside the body.

Colitis is the inflammation of the lining of the large intestine. Its first signs are not feeling well, vague discomfort in the abdomen, and mild diarrhea or constipation. As the disease progresses symptoms like bleeding from the rectum, fever, loss of appetite, and weight loss develop.

Hernia is the protrusion of part of the abdominal contents through a defect in the wall of the abdominal cavity. The most common site for a hernia is the groin, but they occur in other places as well.

Hemorrhoids (piles) are enlarged veins around the anus. External piles can be seen and felt below the anus. Internal piles may also occur. Hemorrhoids are a common cause of bleeding from the rectum.

Diet

An increased fiber content in the form of whole grains and vegetables is essential in the healthy function of the large intestine. Numerous scientific studies have shown that a high protein, high fat diet, low in fiber and complex carbohydrates, leads to many of the diseases of modern people including cancer, heart and vessel diseases, and digestive disorders. Whole cereal grains such as oats, millet, barley, rye, corn, brown rice, buckwheat, and whole wheat are the most abundant sources of fiber. Vegetables, beans, and fruits also supply good amounts. Minerals and nutrients found in sea-weed are an important addition to the diet. Fermented foods such as miso soup and pickles add valuable enzymes to aid in both digestion and assimilation.

The avoidance of congesting and excessive heat or cold producing foods should be observed. These include beef, eggs, chicken, sugar, honey, milk and its products, alcohol, and the nightshade family of vegetables (potato, tomato, eggplant, bell pepper, and tobacco), as well as curry and spices. Raw or cold foods encourage diarrhea in people with poorly functioning intestines.

Shiatsu

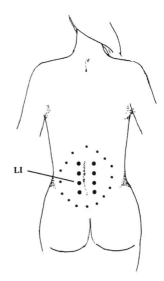

A full shiatsu treatment will strengthen the body and digestion. Specifically, shiatsu application on the back and abdomen can be done.

Have the receiver lie face down. With the heel of one hand press and rub in a circular movement, thus warming the area. This is to be applied in the mid-to-lower back from T_{12} to the sacrum.

Then, while standing over the receiver, press with the thumbs down the channel near the spine beginning at L_2 to the sacrum. Hold each point for 3-5 seconds; repeat several times.

Have the receiver turn over and massage the abdominal area. With the heel of the hand, stimulate circulation with a circular motion of the palm. Next place both hands flat on the abdomen and push and pull, somewhat like kneading bread. Then with the tips of the fingers together, one hand on top of the other, press directly down on the abdomen, while exhaling together with the receiver. Begin in the pit of the stomach moving downward toward the waist and then continue in a circular direction around the inside of the abdominal cavity. Move from one point to the next, as if the abdomen was the face of a clock and you were moving from one number to the next. (See full treatment section for complete description of abdominal massage.)

Diarrhea is the frequent passage of loose stools. For infants, diarrhea is rare if they are breast fed. In bottle fed babies, it is usually due to unsuitable feeding (such as too much fat or sugar), or to gastroenteritis, which is an infection of the bowel. It can be serious in young babies, and quickly leads to dehydration on account of the fluid loss from both diarrhea and vomiting. Urgent treatment is necessary.

In older children and adults, diarrhea can be of two main kinds: sudden onset, which is caused from unsuitable food, such as unripe or too much fruit; or food poisoning—food contaminated by bacteria. Along with diarrhea there can be nausea, vomiting, colic, and fever. Dehydration can follow due to loss of fluids. Drugs and medicines may also cause diarrhea. Long-term diarrhea may be related to having had certain operations such as those of the stomach or intestine. Crohn's disease causes symptoms of diarrhea, malnutrition, and malabsorption. This is usually found in the 20-30 age group. Intestinal parasites can cause diarrhea; amebic dysentery is one such common source. Additionally, more serious troubles can cause diarrhea; they are: diverticular disease of the large intestine, ulcerative colitis, intestine cancer, allergies, poisons and drugs, and irritable bowel syndrome.

Weakness in the stomach or intestines, as well as chilling in the lumbar and leg regions, causes poor digestion. Improperly digested food stimulates the mucous membranes of the intestine, thus speeding up the peristalsis and causing the contents to pass rapidly through the system before liquid is adequately absorbed. Therefore, the contents reach the rectum in a more liquid state than is normal. There are other stimuli which can create imbalances in the autonomic nervous system causing the intestine to speed the transportation time through the bowel before all the liquid has been reabsorbed. In both cases the end result is diarrhea.

In all cases of intestinal trouble, diet is the first adjustment which must be made.

Stomach

stomachache

nausea

overweight

lack of appetite (anorexia)

indigestion

ulcer

The stomach is the principle organ of digestion. It is the largest and most expansive part of the digestive tract. Located in the upper abdominal cavity, the stomach receives and digests food. It is lined with mucous membranes which protect the stomach itself from the strong digestive acids like hydrochloric acid which it secretes. Stomachache, which usually is pain in the abdomen not the stomach, can have a variety of sources (see illustration). Nausea is the feeling which usually comes before vomiting, and is often described as "feeling queasy." The sensation of nausea may be accompanied by a sinking feeling in the stomach, by a feeling of

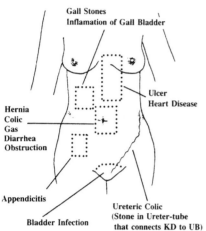

Abdominal Pain

Gall Stones
Inflamation of Gall Bladder

Ulcer
Heart Disease

Hernia
Colic
Gas
Diarrhea
Obstruction

Appendicitis

Bladder Infection

Ureteric Colic
(Stone in Ureter-tube
that connects KD to UB)

weakness, by dizziness, by perspiration, and by excessive salivation. The person will often look pale and sweaty. Nausea may also be part of motion sickness. Modern medicine says that nausea can arise from a disorder in the vagus nerve, which runs from the head down the side of the neck to the front of the chest. Traditional Chinese medicine recognizes the relationship between the pancreas and the stomach. Pancreas disorders can affect the stomach, causing problems with that organ.

Shiatsu

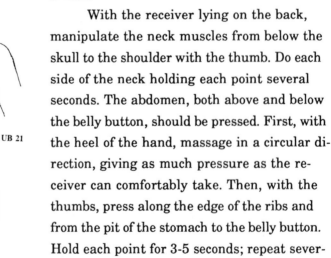

UB 21

With the receiver lying on the back, manipulate the neck muscles from below the skull to the shoulder with the thumb. Do each side of the neck holding each point several seconds. The abdomen, both above and below the belly button, should be pressed. First, with the heel of the hand, massage in a circular direction, giving as much pressure as the receiver can comfortably take. Then, with the thumbs, press along the edge of the ribs and from the pit of the stomach to the belly button. Hold each point for 3-5 seconds; repeat several times. Then place one palm of the hand directly on the belly and the other hand on top of the first hand. Breathing in and out at the same time as the receiver, press down on an exhalation. Repeat at least 10 times. (See full abdominal massage section for details.)

On the leg, press acupoints ST 36 and on the inside of the forearm press acupoint HG 6. Both these points are extremely effective for stomach and nausea complaints.

Have the receiver turn over. On the back, press the back acupoints from T_9 to T_{12}.

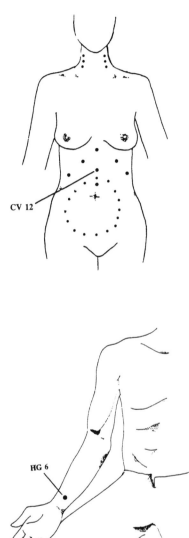

Moxibustion

Moxibustion is very effective for most stomach troubles. Raw or cold foods and beverages will aggravate nausea and stomachache. The warmth of moxa burning brings immediate relief.

Warm each point for 2-5 minutes. ST 36, HG 6, CV 12, UB 21.

Special Foods

For nausea, lack of appetite, indigestion, and ulcer—prepare Kuzu-Umeboshi drink.

---

overeating

Excessive eating is caused by nutritional imbalances or emotional states. Eating the macrobiotic diet, which is rich in nutrients, will satisfy the body's physical requirement. Regular shiatsu treatments with its healing touch will help meet the emotional requirement. Eating more calories than your body needs for its day to day activities will eventually create an overweight condition. Being conscious of the types of foods that are eaten is the first step in getting the diet under control. Cheese and desserts are rich in calories compared with whole grains and vegetables, which are less fatty. Your emotional state and your ideas surrounding food and eating are equally important. Both the foods that you eat and your relationship with eating must be looked into. If throughout the day you dislike your living or working situation and at night you reward yourself for having made it through another day with several large bowls of vanilla ice cream with chocolate sauce and toasted walnuts on top, just trying not to eat ice cream will be a very difficult task. If, on the other hand, you realize your living or work situation is not promoting your happiness, you can either change the situation or at the very least reward yourself with activity instead of food. In other words, reward yourself by visiting friends, going to the theatre, or any other pleasurable activity instead of eating. In this way not only will you lose weight, but your self image will improve.

Acupuncture or a plastic acu-clip, placed in the ear worn like an earring, can reduce the urge to eat.

---

motion sickness

For motion sickness—although it sounds strange, both the eating of salted plums (*umeboshi*) and the placing of one taped on the navel are beneficial in treating this condition.

Pancreas/Spleen

The pancreas is a large gland situated at the back of the abdominal cavity, behind the stomach and between the duodenum

and the spleen. The pancreas has two functions. It produces various enzymes necessary for digestion and it produces hormones
which are released into the bloodstream.
These include insulin and glucogon, which
are essential to normal carbohydrate metabolism, as well as newly discovered hormones related to digestion.

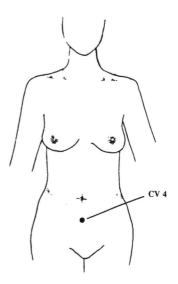

In traditional Chinese medicine, the
functions of both the pancreas and the spleen
are considered as one system. That is why
we have grouped pancreas and spleen together here.

The spleen is an organ also lying within the abdominal cavity. It is situated under the edge of the ribs on the left side. Its size and
shape are about the same as your cupped hand. The spleen is the
largest organ in the lymphatic system, which includes the lymph
nodes located throughout the body. Blood flows through the spleen
where blood-cleansing cells are located. Old
blood cells, abnormal cells, and foreign particles in the blood are removed from circulation here. Blood flow leaves the spleen and
continues on to the liver.

The spleen also plays an important
role in the production of antibodies, which are
part of the body's resistance to infection.

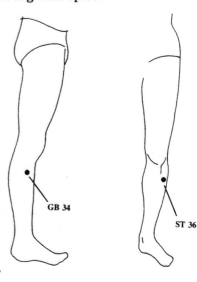

---

hypoglycemia
diabetes
dizziness

135

The level of sugar in the blood, mainly in the form of glucose, is carefully controlled by a variety of mechanisms, including the action of insulin and other hormones. In Diabetes Mellitus, this control is defective and the blood sugar level rises beyond normal limits. This condition is called hyperglycemia. Measurement of the blood sugar level provides a confirmation test for diabetes.

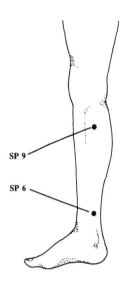

SP 9

SP 6

When too much insulin is in the blood, an excessive fall in the blood sugar level occurs, giving rise to hypoglycemia. Missing a meal will also lower blood sugar levels. Some symptoms associated with this condition are feeling unwell, anxiety, dizziness, panic, hunger and restlessness, palpitations, excessive sweating, flushing of the face, abnormal behavior, and fainting.

The aim of treatment is to strengthen the pancreas so that it respond accurately to the normal fluctuations of sugar in the blood.

Diabetics taking insulin must *not* stop the medication all at once. A regimen of diet, exercise, and shiatsu for adult onset diabetes can be successful so that at some point insulin may be discontinued. However, this must be supervised.

Childhood onset diabetes it is more difficult to cure, but this treatment may lower the amount of insulin required to maintain stable blood sugar levels.

Improper eating patterns and allowing yourself to get overly tired will exhaust the pancreas and increase insulin dosage for diabetics. The key to success is to eat well, exercise, and lead a well regulated life.

Diet

Excessively oily, fatty, and sweet foods should be avoided. Choose a diet high in complex rather than simple sugars. These are found in whole grain products, which should be about 50-60% of the foods consumed. Millet can be used regularly. It can be mixed and cooked with brown rice in a 50-50 or 80-20 ratio of rice to millet. The grains should be cooked with a pinch of quality seasalt. A variety of greens and root vegetables can be used including: kale, cabbage, daikon radish, turnip, carrot and its top, watercress, onion, and sweet squash. A special dish of Squash-Aduki bean-Kombu seaweed can be cooked and taken regularly. The enzyme action of pickles can be beneficial and should be included on a daily basis in the diet. Fruits should be avoided as much as possible. Sweet desserts made from carrot, squash, pumpkin, etc., with a dash of brown rice syrup or malted grain syrup can be used occasionally.

In the case of either hypoglycemia or diabetes, it is better to eat small quantities of food 4-5 times a day rather than to eat large meals less frequently. The last meal of the day should be at least 3 hours before bedtime.

Shiatsu

A complete shiatsu treatment is the most effective way to strengthen the body and the immune system. The spleen and stomach channels in the acupuncture system travel on the legs, therefore the legs should be massaged vigorously, particularly acupoints GB 34 and ST 36 on the outside of the leg, and acupoints SP 9 and SP 6 on the inside of the leg. Additionally, shiatsu on the back between T_9 and L_2 near the spine will stimulate the pancreas and spleen. These points should be held for 3-5 seconds and repeated several times. The neck area, especially the 2 indented points near the skull (GB 20) are helpful in dispersing dizziness.

Moxibustion

Warming several points will enhance the immune system and help to regulate sugar metabolism. Heat each point for 2-5 minutes. Use ST 36, SP 6, UB 20, UB 21 and CV 4

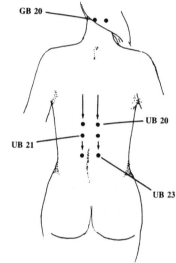

AIDS

Acquired immune deficiency syndrome is a severe breakdown in the body's protective system. Someone with AIDS doesn't have the normal immune protective factors that fight off common bacteria and viruses. Such common maladies as colds and flu can be very dangerous for someone with deficient immune responses. Without major changes in the immune system function, AIDS is fatal.

Diet

A very careful approach to the macrobiotic diet must be adhered to in order to overcome the severe debility of AIDS. Included in the diet should be 50-60% whole cereal grains, without the use of flour products, such as cakes, cookies, breads, pancakes, etc. Miso soup 1-2 times per day should include seaweed and onions as well as other vegetables. Cooked vegetables should be used from root, squash and leafy green categories—no raw salads. Beans cooked with seaweed especially kombu, should be taken in small volume (5-15 %). Nuts and fruits should be avoided temporarily. Also avoid meat, chicken, eggs, oil, and sugars (see diet section).

Shiatsu

Regular shiatsu treatments will stimulate the important natural defenses of the body in preventing AIDS. For someone with AIDS, the treatment must be adjusted according to their condition. If they are strong, then a vigorous treatment can be given. If they are weak, then a light shiatsu or palm healing can be given.

Moxibustion and Acupuncture

Both these therapies can be used to enhance the immune system. Moxa can be given at home. Warm acupoints: ST 36, SP 6, LI 4, CV 4, CV 6, and UB 23.

Acupuncture must be administered by a professional.

---

cancer

Cancer is most easily understood as the development and subsequent spread throughout the body of cells from a malignant tumor. The unique feature of cancer cells is their readiness to multiply outside their organ of origin. The cells can be carried by the blood stream or the lymph system to other parts of the body where they grow. This growth can eventually destroy the healthy tissue that surrounds it. In the early stages cancerous tumors may be indistinguishable from benign or harmless growths such as warts, moles or cysts. Some warning signals of the possible presence of a malignant tumor include: blood in the urine or feces, abnormal bleeding from the vagina, change in regularity of menstrual periods, change in the frequency of bowel movements or in the passing of urine, change in the voice, unexplained weight loss, pain in the chest, coughing up blood, sudden onset of shortness of breath, or a persistent cough.

All of these symptoms may be associated with a disease other than cancer, but may be signs of an early cancer also.

At the request of the United States Senate, a report entitled, *Diet, Nutrition, and Cancer,* was released by the National Academy of Sciences in 1982. It recommends changes in the American diet which they feel will reduce the incidence of cancer. The following are the recommendations that they made:

1. Reduce consumption of fats, both saturated and unsaturated, to 30% of your calorie intake. Most Americans eat over 40% fat in milk products, oils, beef and chicken. This change could reduce the incidence of breast, prostate, and colon cancers.

2. Eat more whole grains, vegetables, and fruits. This advice is given because these foods either contain good amounts of recommended vitamins, such as C or A, or because they contain a certain type of "cancer protection" chemistry. There is a specific warning not to take vitamin or mineral supplements to reduce the risk of cancer because many of them (vitamin D, A, selenium, fluorine) are toxic if taken in large amounts.

3. Minimize the consumption of cured foods such as bacon, ham, bologna, salami, hot dogs, sausage, corned beef, and cured fish. The nitrates and nitrites contained within these foods can form powerful carcinogens called nitrosamines.

4. If you drink alcohol, do so in moderation, particularly if you smoke cigarettes. Alcohol may make it easier for carcinogens to get into your body. It is strongly associated with cancers of the mouth, voice box and esophagus (the passage between the mouth and stomach). Smokers who drink have a greater chance of getting cancers in these areas than smokers who do not drink.

Cancer is a very serious illness. Standard medical treatments include surgery, radiotherapy (radiation), and chemotherapy (use of cell killing drugs). Even with such strong and powerful treatments, no one can say that cancer is easy to cure. Cancer will affect one in three Americans within their lifetime. It is the second leading cause of death. The link between diet and cancer is growing. Prevention of cancer is the cure of the future. Many people have cured their cancers with the macrobiotic diet; however, don't wait for cancer to develop to begin the diet. Follow common sense and prevent cancer with proper lifestyle which includes the macrobiotic diet, exercise, full deep breathing, positive mental outlook, and a vitality and enjoyment of life.

Cancer Prevention Diet

This macrobiotic diet includes : whole grains, soup, vegetable dishes, beans and sea vegetables, and perhaps—depending on the individual—fish, fruit, desserts, and snacks. Of course, beverages can be consumed by all. (See *Cancer Prevention Diet* by Michio Kushi with Alex Jack.)

Shiatsu

Someone with cancer can receive shiatsu. However, care must be taken not to overstimulate the individual with too strong a treatment as this may encourage cancer cells to move from one part of the body to another. The cancer site must not be massaged. For example, if colon cancer is present, then do not massage the abdomen. Instead palm healing can be done on the cancer area.

Palm Healing

Gently place the palms directly on the troubled area and hold for some time while you breath slow and deep. This is a palm healing technique. No physical force is used, only the laying on of hands. This is helpful in dealing with pain and promoting healing.

allergy

hay fever

Many people suffer from the symptoms associated with allergies. Allergy is the mechanism through which symptoms are caused by sensitivity to an allergen (allergy causing substance). Allergy is the cause of hay fever and hives (urticaria) and underlies many cases of asthma and eczema.

Allergic reactions are exaggerations of the body's normal immune responses to bacteria and viruses and their toxins. The normal immune response is designed to destroy bacteria and neutralize their toxins. The allergic response causes symptoms rather than protecting against them.

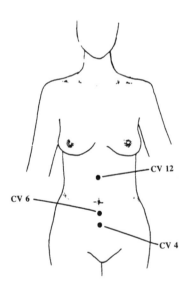

The most common sites for allergic reactions are the respiratory tract and the skin. It is the body's own histamine reaction to foreign matter that creates the symptoms of hay fever such as sneezing and eye-watering from swelling and inflammation around the eyes and the nasal mucous membranes. In the lungs the small air passages spasms causing asthma; in the skin the response causes swelling and irritation. Allergy can affect the digestive system by damaging the lining, causing chronic diarrhea.

Many allergy symptoms are caused by yeast infections. Yeast are single cell fungi which belong to the vegetable kingdom. Yeast is found all around us. *Candida albicans* normally lives in your body and more especially in your intestines and other parts of your digestive tract. They live on the mucous membranes of the digestive tract and vagina. So do billions of friendly germs. Unfriendly bacteria, viruses, allergens, and other enemies also find their way into these and other membrane-lined passageways and cavities. But when your immune system is strong, they aren't able to break through into your deeper tissues or blood stream and make you sick.

When you take antibiotics, especially repeatedly, you wipe out the friendly bacteria (especially in the digestive tract). Since yeasts aren't harmed they spread out and grow in other parts of your body. When yeasts multiply, they put out toxins which circulate through your body and make you sick. These toxins weaken your immune system. Other factors also adversely affect your immune system leading to more allergies, infections, and antibiotics.

Antibiotics, especially broad-spectrum antibiotics, kill friendly germs while they're killing enemies. This allows yeast (*candida albicans*) to multiply. Diets rich in sugar and the use of birth control pills, cortisone, and other drugs also stimulate yeast growth.

When your immune system is weak, you're apt to feel "sick all over" and develop yeast and/or fungus infections of the skin, nails, or vagina. You may also become more susceptible to viral, bacterial and other infections, and develop mold, chemical, food and other allergies, intolerances, and sensitivities. You may also develop other health disorders, including hives, psoriasis, arthritis, Crohn's disease, or multiple sclerosis.

You can suspect yeast as the cause of your allergy if you have taken antibiotics in the past; experience fatigue, depression, and headache frequently; have digestive and sex organ problems; and feel "sick all over." Confirmation of this suspicion is particularly likely if, after some weeks, the elimination of sugar, yeasted products, fruit, and milk products makes you feel better.

Allergy treatment is aimed at strengthening the body's immune system and dealing with symptoms that exist during that process.

Diet

Diet is the foundation of a healthy body and a strong immune system. Excess protein from animal sources such as beef, lamb and pork; sugars; excessive fried and oily snack foods like potato chips; and refined and chemicalized foods can contribute to lowering the immune system. Being exposed to environmental contaminants and chemicals put severe stress on the natural defense mechanisms of the body. Lack of adequate exercise or breathing of fresh air prevents the body from becoming strong. Regular exercise increases body resistance.

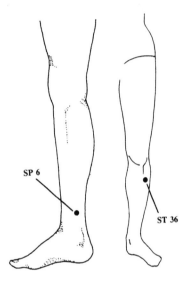

The standard macrobiotic diet will aid in the strengthening process of the immune system. Depending on the severity of symptoms, fruit, fruit juices, fried foods, and the use of flour products should be eliminated or minimized. If your symptoms are severe, then the elimination of luxury items such as fruit is necessary. If symptoms are not very bad, then small amounts of cooked fruit may be tolerated.

In the case of allergy caused by yeast infection (*candida albicans*) you must be especially attentive to the diet.

Food You Can Eat

All fresh vegetables, fish, water, unprocessed nuts, seeds and oils, whole grains (not enriched) such as millet, brown rice, old fashioned oats, barley. One salted plum (umeboshi) per day is useful.

Foods to Avoid

Processed and packaged foods, condiments, yeasted bread

and pastries, mushrooms and truffles, milk and its products, coffee and tea, yeast, alcoholic beverages, all fruit, fruit juices, malt products, dried and candied fruits, processed and smoked meats, luncheon meats, sugar and sugar containing foods.

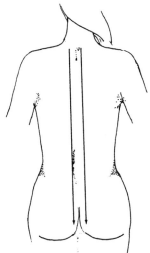

Shiatsu

Regular shiatsu treatments are helpful with allergies. Special attention should be paid to the head and sinus area. The back area, from the shoulders down to the waist, near the spine should be pressed with the thumbs. (See page 77, for complete details on technique.)

Ginger Compress

Compresses placed on the face and sinus area, as well as the abdominal region, will help with the congestion symptoms that accompany allergies. Warm each area for 10-20 minutes.

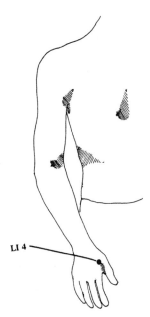

Moxibustion and Acupuncture

Strengthening the immune system with heat applications will enhance the effectiveness of the macrobiotic diet when allergic symptoms are present.

Warm the following acupoints for 2-5 minutes: ST 36, SP 6, CV 4, CV 6, CV 12, and LI 4.

Acupuncture is effective, but must be done by a professional.

bruising easily

A bruise (hematoma) is a swelling composed of blood which has escaped from an injured, diseased, or abnormally fragile vessel into the tissue. Someone who bruises easily has weak vessels. This can be caused by a variety of factors. Among them are lack of exercise and—particularly—the eating of sugars, chemicals, preservatives, fruits, and fruit juices.

To alleviate this condition the standard macrobiotic diet including miso soup and mineral rich sea vegetables is helpful.

When you bruise yourself, immediately rub the affected area with your thumb or palm in a vigorous circular motion. This will minimize the size and tenderness of the bruise.

Heart

hypertension
hypotension
irregular heartbeat
racing heartbeat (tachycardia)
slow heart beat (brachycardia)
excessive pounding of the heart (palpitation)
tightness in the chest (angina)
hardening of the arteries (arteriosclerosis)

The symptoms of heart disease arise from failure of the arteries, which supply blood to the heart muscle itself, to deliver oxygen to the heart muscle. The result can be angina pectoris, which is a deep, aching, crushing or viselike pain in the chest, radiating perhaps to the arm, or the neck and jaw. It is fairly common in men in their forties and older whose arteries have been seriously narrowed by atherosclerosis (hardening in the arteries). A complete blockage of the artery causes a heart attack (myocardial infarction).

Reasons for heart disease have been investigated all around the world. The highest incidence is in Finland, where both blood fat levels and blood pressures are unusually high. Smoking, excessive alcohol consumption, stress, lack of exercise, and obesity greatly increase the risks of developing heart disease. However, dietary factors such as high fat and cholesterol consumption seem to be of greater importance. For example, the Japanese male smokes and drinks as much and is subjected to as much stress as his American counterpart, but he has much lower blood cholesterol levels, and rarely has coronary heart disease. The Japanese diet is much lower in beef, eggs, oil, and dairy products. It relies more on grains, vegetables and fish.

It is widely recognized that heart disease can result from overindulgence and can only be prevented by people themselves. There is a strong relationship between the heart, lungs, and kidneys. As blood pressure increases, breathing is affected and breathlessness may be present. Chronic bronchitis and emphysema lessen the lung's ability to adequately exchange oxygen for carbon dioxide. Under these conditions, the function of the kidneys is impaired, with retention of salt and water and an increase in blood volume. All in all, symptoms affecting the heart, lungs, and/or kidneys cause additional strain on other organs until, in severe cases, either the heart or the kidneys fail and death follows. Fortunately, however, heart disease is preventable with a combination of diet and exercise.

The principles of natural healing are based on balance. When a condition or an organ is either in excess (hyper) or in

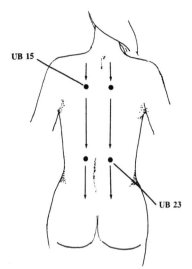

deficiency (hypo), our treatment aim is to re-establish harmony. The body is capable of making appropriate adjustments and correcting our imbalanced conditions. Therefore for both hypertension and hypotension, our shiatsu treatment is approximately the same. If the heart is beating too fast or too slow our treatment is about the same. Our body's adjustment mechanism, following natural patterns is the source of healing.

Shiatsu

The most effective method for any aspect of heart disease is to give a complete shiatsu treatment. In general however, attention to the heart (HT) and heart governor (HG) channels on the arms is effective.

The area on the back between the shoulder blades near the spine (T_3-T_7) can be pressed.

An abdominal massage (see pages 103-105, shiatsu section for details) and shiatsu on the lower back in the kidney region is helpful (T_{12}-L_4).

Moxibustion

Warming several acupoints help to regulate the heart rhythm as well as the kidneys. Heat each acupoint for 2-5 minutes. LI 4, LI 11, LU 9, CV 12, KD 3, UB 15, UB 23, SP 9. Choose from 3-5 acupoints, alternating with each treatment. Treat every 2-3 days until symptoms subside.

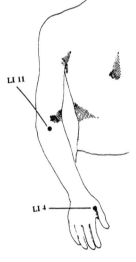

Diet

Proper eating is the single most important factor in both preventing and curing heart disease and the symptoms associated with it. The standard macrobiotic diet, which is low in fats and sugars, and high in complex carbohydrates, vitamins, and minerals, is the best approach to a healthy heart. (See diet section for details.)

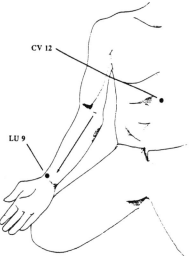

Exercise

For those concerned with overall physical fitness, the ideal exercise is one which involves as many muscles as possible. Walking, jogging, running, swimming and almost any outdoor sport will meet this end.

If exercise is to have its most beneficial effect on the heart and lungs, it must work them at near their maximum capability. You can measure your capability by measuring your pulse rate. The basic guide is that the pulse should not be allowed to rise over 200 minus your age in years. Therefore a 35 year old person would have a maximum pulse rate of 165 beats/ minute (200-35=165). Someone who is totally unfit should add another 20-30 on to his/her age for the first few weeks of the training program. Taking the pulse while exercising will inform you if you should increase or decrease your effort. The pulse rate will serve as a guide to the effects of exercise in improving physical fitness. As strength is increasing, your routine of the same exercises should not force the pulse rate up as it did

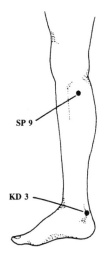

in the past. In other words, the same set of exercises will have a decreased pulse rate over time. In practice, most people find that 40-60 minutes a week is the minimum to maintain reasonably good fitness. This is divided into 3 sessions of 20 minutes. Regular exercise should become an enjoyable part of your lifestyle. The movement itself should be rewarding enough so that on skipped days you will feel like you have missed an indispensable part of the day.

Small Intestine

inability to assimilate nourishment from food

anemia

The functions of the small intestine are digestion and absorption of the liquid contents from the stomach. These contents are alkaline. Just before entering the small intestine two important digestive juices are added. They are bile from the liver (which is alkaline and neutralizes the acid contents from the stomach as well as digests and breaks down fat particles into smaller parts) and pancreatic juice which comes from the pancreas. This juice acts on carbohydrates, fats, and proteins in food. It too is alkaline.

The absorption of digested food takes place entirely in the small intestine through the capillary vessels and the lymphatics found on the surface of the small intestine walls. These products are carried by the portal vein to the liver, where more changes take place.

Shiatsu

A complete shiatsu treatment will enhance the functions of the digestive organs. The stimulus of shiatsu encourages movement and promotes the elimination of intestinal stagnation. Abdominal shiatsu is appropriate. (See pages 103-105, shiatsu section.)

Ginger Compress

Hot compresses placed directly on the abdomen over the umbilicus promote nutrient absorption. Do the compress treatment for 15-20 minutes. Repeat everyday for 2 weeks. Rest one week, then repeat for another 2 weeks.

Diet

The macrobiotic diet with its high vitamin and mineral content promotes positive bacteria growth inside the intestines. Antibiotics, sugars, and other refined foods destroy the beneficial bacteria necessary for proper absorption.

The inclusion of fermented foods such as miso, pickles, and natural whole grain sourdough bread will furnish positive bacteria sources. Small portions of seaweed supply minerals necessary to keep the small intestine alkaline.

Properly functioning spleen, small intestine, and bone marrow insure enough red blood cell production. Therefore clean intestines (cleansed daily by the fiber in whole grains) are essential so that the food nutrients can enter the body to keep systems working. The sweet taste of cooked carrots, parsnips, and onions affect the spleen to make quality red blood cells. This is your protection against anemia.

To treat anemia include miso soup daily. Cooked green leafy vegetables should be included also. The table seasoning *Tekka* can be used—1 teaspoon/day.

Anemia has been studied using garlic as the treatment. In one study, after eight weeks of treatment with garlic extract or cooked garlic, there was substancial improvement in the hemoglobin content of the red blood cell.

Many times the anemia connected with cancer is caused by the toxins of the cancer. In this case charcoal can be taken to remove the toxins. Take one tablespoon of charcoal mixed with 4-6 ounces of water, 3 times each day. Charcoal can be purchased at natural foods stores or you can make your own by charring any vegetable food and pulverizing it. The pits of the salted plum (*umeboshi*) have traditionally been used for this purpose.

Heart Governor/Triple Heater

In addition to the body's ten major organs, traditional Chinese medicine recognizes the usefulness of two functions. These functions were given the names heart governor and triple heater. They are paired like the other organs.

The heart governor is considered the first line of defense for the heart. It functions much the same as the heart.

The triple heater helps with the administration of energy and the fluid metabolism of the body. It coordinates the functions of the three spaces of the trunk. The upper space helps the stomach take in and digest food. The middle space helps the small intestine absorb and transfer the essence of food for body energy and nutrition. The function of the lower space is to help the large intestine and the bladder eliminate waste. From this it can be seen that these functions relate to all the other organs.

Problems in the circulation of energy in these two channels can be seen as circulation trouble, cold hands and feet, body temperature troubles such as too hot or too cold, immune troubles, swelling and water retention, digestive disorders, mental disorders, and so forth.

Urinary System
Kidney/Urinary Bladder

---

infection
inability to hold urine (incontinence)
bedwetting (enuresis)
kidney stone

The urinary system consists of the kidneys, which secrete urine; the ureters, the passages through which urine travels from the kidney to the bladder; the urinary bladder, which acts as a reservoir; and the urethra, the passage tube through which urine flows from the bladder to outside of the body.

The kidneys regulate water balance. They also regulate the concentration of salts in the blood, as well as the excretion of waste products and any excess salts.

The volume of urine passed each day varies with the volume of fluid drunk, but about one to two quarts is average. Volume of urine passed increases when excess protein is taken, in order to provide the fluid necessary to carry urea (a waste product from protein digestion) away in a solution. That is why doctors instruct those on a diet high in meat, eggs, and cheese to drink "plenty of fluids." Normal urine is a light color, like light beer, and is slightly acid (pH 6). Normally we should pass urine four to five times per day—more often depletes the body of minerals.

The most common kidney ailment which is surgically treated is kidney (renal) stones. The formation of stones in the kidney can cause great damage. They can also be formed in the bladder or may pass from the kidney to the bladder. As the bladder contracts to pass urine, the stone is pressed against the bladder wall causing intense pain. Infection can result from this condition, as well as the inability to hold urine. Excruciating pain and blood in the urine are signs of stones. Their removal does not guarantee a cure, according to medical sources. However it will deal with the immediate pain. Preventive diet is the only way to reduce the risks of recurrence.

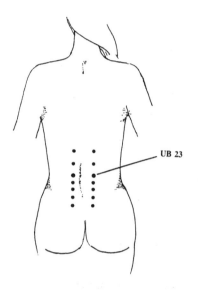

UB 23

Urinary stones usually form as a result of abnormally high levels of calcium or metabolism problems. The combination of high calcium dairy products and certain vegetables such as spinach, chard, and tomato (high in oxalic acid) acts to form calcium oxalates, the most common materials found in stones.

In the case of kidney stone and infection, prevention via diet is important. It is possible for small stones to dissolve and pass out of the body; however, some large stones can form in irregular shapes within the kidney. These irregular shaped stones will not pass and, if they are painful, must be removed. A prudent macrobiotic diet will lessen the formation of all stones.

Shiatsu

For all kidney disorders, including swelling, water retention, inability to hold and pass urine, and bedwetting, shiatsu therapy can stimulate the system to function more efficiently.

Have the receiver lie face down. Stand over the person and ask him or her to breath in and out, as you do the same. On each exhalation press the area near the spine from T_{12}-L_5 with the thumbs. Press and hold the acupoints that make the two parallel lines of the urinary bladder channel. Press these acupoints several times.

Use barefoot shiatsu and walk on the soles of the inturned feet with your feet. Press the hips, upper thighs, and calves with the foot. Do the leg stretches. (See leg part of complete shiatsu section.)

Have the receiver turn over and lie face up. Massage the toes and press the bottoms of the feet with your thumb. Press around the ankles thoroughly. (See page 91, leg section in shiatsu section.)

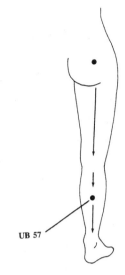

UB 57

Moxibustion

Use moxibustion on several acupoints. This stimulates the bladder and the kidney. Warm each acupoint for 2-5 minutes.

UB 23, UB 57, KD 3, ST 36

Diet

Our daily diet should supply enough calcium as well as other minerals and vitamins. However, some people receive more than enough and, with the addition of certain vegetables or because of some metabolic abnormalities, kidney or bladder stones form. In addition to a standard macrobiotic diet, shiitake mushrooms and radish (especially daikon radish) can be eaten to dissolve stones and clean the blood so as to prevent future formations. Meat and dairy products produce uric acid during digestion; this acid is associated with stone formation. It is best to avoid these foods.

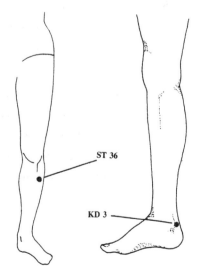

ST 36

KD 3

Reproductive System

The development of the reproductive organs is interesting. Early in embryonic development, germ cells of the testis in the male and of the ovary in the female appear. Sex therefore is determined from the very earliest days but sex characteristics cannot be recognized. At adolescence, these germ cells develop along with the changes which determine the sex qualities and characteristics of the male and female. The female reproductive organs are located in the pelvic region inside the body while the male organs are found mainly outside the pelvis.

The whole reproductive system goes through several changes in a lifetime. The first major change is puberty. This appears at ten to fourteen years and, in girls, is marked by the beginning of menstruation. The uterus and vagina enlarge, while the breasts enlarge with increase of fat and blood vessels. Later the secondary sexual characteristics appear. The curves of the body develop and fat tissue rounds off the contours of her limbs, with the appearance of hair in the underarm and pubic regions. The pelvis also widens. There are further important changes that take place as the girl matures mentally and emotionally through adolescence to womanhood.

In boys, puberty is a little later. It is characterized by deepening of the voice, enlargement of the sex organs, and the appearance of body and facial hair.

Further changes happen at the menopause period of a woman's life which occurs at about forty-five to fifty years of age, but may be earlier or later. Menstruation ceases. The ovaries become smaller and their secretions cease.

irregular menstruation
lack of menstruation (amenorrhea)
painful or difficult menstruation (dysmenorrhea)
pre-menstrual syndrome (PMS)
menopause problems

The incidence of menstrual difficulty is extraordinarily common. The normal female cycle is disrupted from its average period of 28 days by a number of disturbing symptoms. Some women do not menstruate while others have extended or severe bleeding. Symptoms during or just before the monthly cycle can include pain in the lower abdomen, pain in the lumbar region, headaches, and nausea. The breasts sometimes swell and are painful. Many women are unable to continue with normal day to day functions and must go to bed and rest.

The symptoms of pre-menstrual syndrome can be even more debilitating than painful menstruation. The symptoms come on one to two weeks before actual menstruation. These can include mental tension, irritability, headache, depression, and edema (swelling). During this time admissions to psychiatric hospitals, suicides, and accidents are all found to occur more frequently for women. Fortunately all of these symptoms are treatable with shiatsu, diet, and increased exercise.

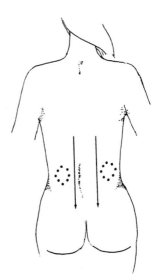

Shiatsu

In many cases the symptoms associated with menstrual difficulties are aggravated by lack of sufficient exercise. A complete shiatsu treatment stimulates circulation and removes the heavy, bloated feeling often associated with these female problems.

Specific shiatsu should be directed to the lower back, abdomen, and the inside of the legs.

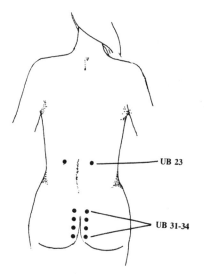

Have the receiver lie face down. Stand over the person and place your thumbs about 1 1/2 inches on each side of the spine, breathe in and out with the receiver and on an exhalation press down, leaning your body weight into the acupoint and hold for 2-5 seconds. Begin this press technique beneath the ribs at T_{12} and continue until the lower end of the tail bone. Repeat each point several times.

With the palm of the hand massage in a circular movement over the kidney area.

Have the receiver turn over. Massage the lower section of the abdomen beneath the navel with the heel of the hand in a circular movement. Use care as this area may be tender and painful to the touch. Give the proper amount of pressure that will increase circulation and yet not create additional pain.

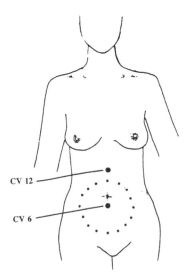

Place one hand, palm down, on the navel and the other hand directly on top. You and the receiver should breathe in a deep full breath and on an exhalation press gently down until you find resistance. Hold for 1-5 seconds. Repeat at least 10 times. Finish by massaging the entire area again with the heel of the hand.

Massage the bottom of the feet and press with your thumb the lines on the inside of the legs. The channels found here are related to the reproductive organs. Many times you will find tenderness around the ankle and just below the knee on the inside. Any tender spots are worth massaging a little extra. Work up and down each line 2-5 times.

Moxibustion

Moxa treatment is very effective in relaxing menstrual cramping and discomfort. Warm each acupoint from 2-5 minutes. Use the following acupoints: on the abdomen—CV 6, CV 12; on the back—UB 23, UB 31-34; on the legs—SP 9, SP 6, KD 3.

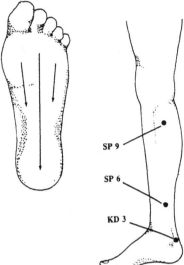

Diet

Foods that retard the circulation of blood and energy should be restricted when menstrual troubles are present. They include: fatty items such as beef, cheese, milk and other dairy products, avocado, potato chips, and other fried, greasy foods. Sugars, honey, and fruit juice should be avoided and, temporarily, fruits as well. Stay away from raw salads and other cold foods which tax digestion and cool down the inside making internal contractions severe and painful.

The diet should include energizing warm foods which will relax excessive muscle contractions. A high fiber diet, taken in the form of whole grains, vegetables, and beans, has the ability to remove excessive estrogen from the body. The phytic acid present in fiber binds excess estrogen, thus removing this substance which is known to increase muscle cramping. This will help to establish the correct ratio of estrogen to progesterone (female hormones made by the ovaries) which is linked to the symptoms of pre-menstrual syndrome.

Miso soup taken daily supplies adequate protein and vitamins including vitamin B$_{12}$. Wakame seaweed and daikon radish (or turnip) added to the soup add a delicious flavor and medicinal qualities.

Ginger Compress

Compresses can be placed on the lower abdomen and/or the lower back, whichever you feel is appropriate. The warm, stimulating effect of the compress will help to alleviate pain rapidly.

Hip Bath

Prepare a hip bath in one of two ways. You may use dried radish leaves (daikon preferred) and place 4-5 bunches in one gallon of water and simmer until the water turns brown. Add this liquid to a full bathtub.

The second method is to add a handful of seasalt to the bathtub.

Once the bath water is prepared, sit with the water level at least up to the waist. Cover the upper part of your body with a towel or blanket. Your body will become very warm and begin to sweat. This takes about 10-20 minutes. Repeat this bath up to 10 days.

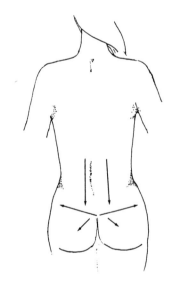

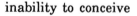

inability to conceive

There are many reasons why there can be difficulty for a couple to conceive and have children. Low sperm count is one condition affecting males, while blocked fallopian tubes or hormonal inbalances can affect the female making conception impossible. The ability to produce children depends on more than physiological readiness. It requires a combination of correctly timed physical and hormonal events, a suitable mental attitude by both partners and many other less understood factors that we can just call luck. The habit of throwing rice after the wedding ceremony is based on ancient "fertility rites."

Yet even though no physical problems can be found that should stop a couple from having children, there are times when conception does not occur. Shiatsu helps to regulate the indidivuals and may be useful.

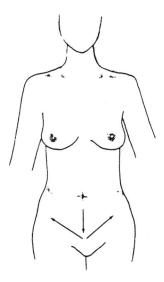

Shiatsu

Have the receiver lie face down. Use thumb pressure to treat the lower back region near the lumber vertebrae. Press around the hip bones and on the buttocks.

Have the receiver turn over onto the back. Massage the lower abdomen. Beneath the navel, press and hold. Move the thumbs down to the pubic bone, press around the pelvic bones.

---

pain during childbirth

For *pain during childbirth,* massage the area near the ankle on the inside of the leg (SP 6). and the area around the back of the hips (same as preceding treatment). The acupoints of the hands (LI 4) are helpful.

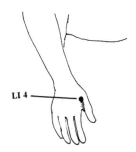

breech position of child before delivery

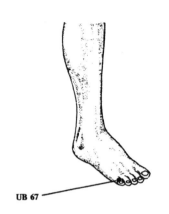

UB 67

Breach position of the fetus can be reversed in a good number of cases. In China, studies have shown that by using moxibustion (see moxibustion section) on one acupoint, the fetus can move to the correct delivery position. This occurs in 90% of woman treated. Moxibustion is applied to UB 67 (Zhiyin) on both feet. The heating is controlled so as not to produce burning pain. It is applied once a day for 15 minutes. Most can be corrected within one to four treatments. Some take up to 10 treatments. It is assumed that stimulation of UB 67 increases secretion of the adrenal cortex which enhances uterine activity. At the time of treatment, the movement of the fetus increases. This favor the automatic correction of the fetal position.

frigidity

impotence

Healthy and enjoyable sexual relations enhance a couple's relationship. Unfortunately, the number of problems connected with the woman's menstrual cycle and the man's prostate and urinary functions interferes greatly with this pleasurable aspect of life, much to the detriment of many relationships.

A full shiatsu treatment is the best method for increasing circulation and balancing the body. The stress of modern living or unknown psychological causes contribute to sexual problems. Accidents and the use of drugs and alcohol can contribute as well. Shiatsu is effective in dealing with these problems.

swollen and tight prostate

prostate pain

difficulty in passing urine

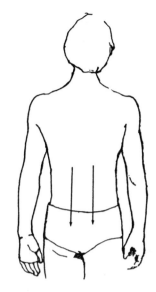

The prostate gland in the male is about the size of a large walnut. It lies below the bladder, surrounding the urethra, and is made up of glands, tubes, and muscle. The prostate secretes a fluid which mingles with the secretion of the testes. When the prostate becomes enlarged, it obstructs the urethra and causes retention of urine.

Diet

A diet high in fat, protein, sugar, and coffee will enlarge the prostate. This is a very common occurrence in men past the age of 45. Treatment is aimed at reducing the size of the prostate and increasing overall body strength.

It is best to avoid the fatty animal foods such as beef, poultry, cheese, milk, and eggs. Not only animal food, but also sugar, honey, chocolate, and all sugary foods should be discontinued. All stimulants including mustard, pepper, curry, mint, peppermint, spices, alcohol, and coffee should be avoided. All vegetables and fruits that cause a swelling effect should be avoided. These include potato, tomato, eggplant, and tropical fruits.

The standard macrobiotic diet should be followed. Dried shiitake mushrooms cooked with carrots or daikon can be eaten

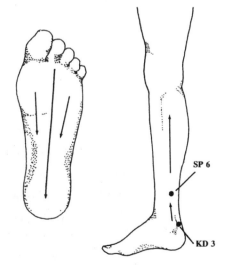

frequently. One or two tablespoons of grated fresh raw daikon or carrot also can be used several times per week as a condiment at meals.

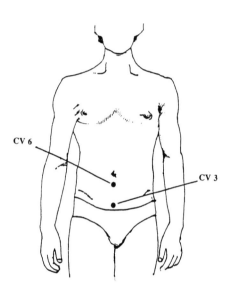

Shiatsu

Have the receiver lie face down. Press the acupoints near the spine on the lower hip region. Repeat this several times. Massage the bottoms of the feet with the thumbs vigorously. Massage up the inside of the legs.

Moxibustion

Heat applied to acupoints CV 3, CV 6, SP 6, KD 3 will bring rapid relief for difficulty in passing urine. Prostate pain is alleviated after 1-5 weeks of consistently eating the macrobiotic diet. It definitely is worth the effort of making the necessary changes in eating.

Liver and Gall Bladder

rib pain (intercostal neuralgia)
gall stone pain
hepatitis
jaundice

The liver and gall bladder system play an important role in maintaining health. The liver is the largest gland in the body, situated in the uppermost part of the abdominal cavity on the right side beneath the diaphragm. It is largely protected by the ribs. The liver develops in the embryo as an outgrowth of the intestine and always retains a close link with the digestive system. We can think of the liver as the largest chemical factory in the body in that it carries out most of the intermediate metabolism. That is, it changes the nutrients absorbed from the small intestine and makes them suitable for use by the body tissues. The liver also modifies waste products and toxic substances to make them suitable for excretion in the bile or the urine. Enzymes in the liver stimulate the production of glycogen (a complex sugar), which is derived from carbohydrate foods such as whole grains and vegetables. This substance is stored temporarily by the liver cells and converted back into glucose (a simple sugar) by enzyme action when needed by the body tissue. Along with this liver function, insulin, a secretion by the pancreas, controls the blood sugar level at the normal level of 80-100 mg/100cc of blood. Some of the materials in bile (a digester of fats) are made in the liver.

When the liver receives the building blocks of protein (amino acids) it separates the nitrogen from the amino acid part. This nitrogen in the form of ammonia is converted into urea (a waste product). Urea is removed from the body by the kidneys and excreted in the urine.

The liver makes substances essential for blood clotting. It also stores and distributes glycogen, fat, vitamins, and iron. The liver also maintains body temperature and protects the body as a whole. As a detoxifier, it removes drugs, alcohol, waste products formed from protein metabolism, and other harmful substances from the blood stream.

The gall bladder is a pear-shaped muscular bag situated on the undersurface of the liver. It is about 3-4 inches in length and holds about two fluid ounces of bile. The gall bladder acts as a storage place for bile. It also serves to concentrate the bile that is stored in it.

Within half an hour of taking food, bile flows into the lower part of the duodenum which connects with the stomach. The flow is not continuous but occurs only when foods enter this lower part. Bile is an alkaline fluid made by the liver cells. Pigments in the bile color the stool. Bile salts digest fats and aid in their absorption.

The liver and gall bladder are subject to various troubles. The liver may be ruptured by injury which can cause serious bleeding. Toxic degeneration and cirrhosis (hardening, sometimes associated with alcohol consumption) affect the liver. Its function is impaired when congestive heart disease, as well as cancer, produces symptoms of jaundice, vomiting, and fluid retention in the abdomen (ascites).

The gall bladder can become infected or can be blocked by the presence of gall stones. Stones in the gall bladder and the cystic duct do not cause jaundice. But when they block the common bile duct, jaundice can occur. If a stone passes down the bile duct it may cause severe pain called biliary colic. Stone production has been linked to excessive cholesterol and calcium in the body.

Diet

Liver trouble is often the result of overeating. Therefore, in treating the liver and gall bladder, it is best to perhaps fast or eat small amounts for a period of time. Also chewing well is important. The food should be liquid by the time it is to be swallowed. When severe pain is present the diet should be restricted to brown rice soup with cooked green leafy vegetables. Salty foods and animal products should be avoided. After several days the diet can be widened to include regular macrobiotic foods, but fish and other animal foods should be avoided until symptoms have subsided.

In the case of jaundice the individual should avoid all dairy foods, eggs, sugar, and oily or greasy foods, and should eat the standard macrobiotic diet. Daikon radish can be eaten daily as it helps to dissolve mucus or fat accumulations in the blood stream and body. The sour flavor enhances the liver's function, therefore foods such as sauerkraut, salted plums (*umeboshi*), plum extract tea, and mugwort tea can be used beneficially. Traditional Oriental medicine has used the extract of clam for treatment of jaundice. This extract is known as "cobicula" and is available in natural food stores.

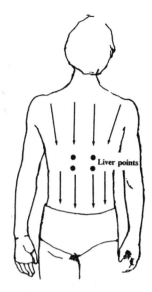

In the case of gall stones, foods which contribute to mucus or fat formation should be discontinued. Beef and cheese are examples of high fat and cholesterol foods. By-products from protein and fat digestion join with calcium to form calcium carbonate and calcium phosphate, these are the major ingredients of gall stones. These hard stones are either formed or lodged in the gall bladder, creating gall bladder pain and inflammation. Fall and winter sweet squashes such as acorn, buttercup, blue hubbard, butternut, and banana can be eaten regularly to help prevent stones from being formed. The passing of a stone can be extremely painful. When the stone begins to move, you can place hot ginger compresses on the painful area and drink several cups of hot twig tea. This will relax the muscles, expand the duct, and allow the stone to pass through more freely. For this condition shiitake mushroom tea can be used as an alternative to twig tea.

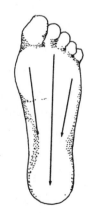

Ginger Compress

In all conditions involving the liver and gall bladder, ginger compress can be used. In the case of a painful and swollen liver, the ginger compress can be followed by a taro potato plaster. If there is water trapped in the abdomen, then the ginger compress can be followed by a buckwheat plaster which can remove this retained fluid.

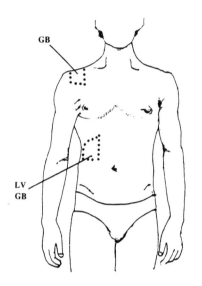

Shiatsu

In Oriental medicine the liver function is to maintain the unrestricted flow of vital energy. When the liver fails in this function we observe depression, irritability, or fits of anger. It is because the liver energy is stagnant and unable to move freely that symptoms arise. Shiatsu is effective in reestablishing the free circulation of vital energy, thereby strengthening the liver.

When possible complete a full shiatsu session.

If you can only apply shiatsu to specific areas, choose the following:

Have the receiver lie face down. Near the spine begin at T_7 and continue until L_4. Do thumb shiatsu pressing down leaning your body weight into the back while the receiver is exhaling. Repeat the two bladder lines which travel down the back. The first line is located 11/2 inches from the vertebrae and the second line is 3 inches away from the spine. You will find several very tender spots at the level of T_9-T_{10} on the back. These are liver acupoints.

Massage the bottoms of the feet and each toe.

Have the receiver lie on the back. The area under the right rib cage is where the liver and gall bladder are located. This area will be tender. The right shoulder and top of the right eye may be tender in the case of gall stones. Press around the liver with the tips of your right hand to evaluate the degree of pain present. If the receiver can tolerate pressure, press with the thumb along the edge of the rib. If the pain is too intense for shiatsu, you can apply palm healing here.

Five Transformations

The interrelatedness of all creation is represented in the Five Transformations. The natural elements of fire, earth, metal, water, and wood are used to explain energy's endless stages. In ancient Asian classics the functions and relationships of the elements were explained. Water and fire are essential in order to eat. Metal and wood are basic tools for carrying out production. And earth is for the growth of everything. These transformations are considered indispensable for the continuity of life. They are used to generalize about everything in the universe and are not limited solely to solid elements.

The five transformation theory is a helpful tool which can unify and clarify formerly unknown relationships within the body. For example, people who are losing head hair and are fearful, may have kidney trouble (see chart on next page). They can be helped by the addition of aduki beans and more green leafy vegetables in the diet. This will strengthen the kidney function.

One element can act as a promoter to another element, e.g., fire can promote earth. At the same time one element can counteract against another element, e.g., fire works against metal (see chart).

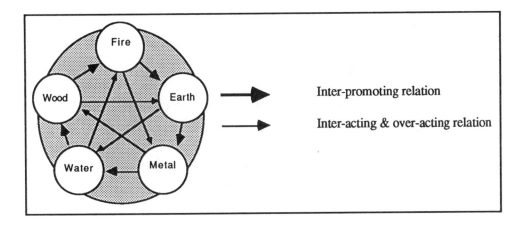

Inter-promoting relation

Inter-acting & over-acting relation

The classification of the five transformations reflects our dependence on nature. It also explains adaptability of both man and nature. The classifications are based on environment, climatic changes, and geographical influences on the human body. Understanding this classification system, one can more easily understand illness and physiology.

Organ	Lung Large Intestine	Spleen/Pancreas Stomach	Heart Small Intestine	Kidney Urinary Bladder	Liver Gall Bladder
Element	Metal	Earth	Fire	Water	Wood
Season	Fall	Late Summer	Summer	Winter	Spring
Flavor	Pungent	Sweet	Bitter	Salty	Sour
Grain	Brown Rice	Millet	Corn	Azuki	Wheat
Vegetable	Onion	Squash	Scallions	Greens	Leeks
Fruit	Peach	Date	Apricot	Chestnut	Plum
Governs	Skin & Body Hair	Flesh	Blood Vessels	Head Hair & Bones	Ligaments & Muscles
Humor	Runny Eyes & Nose	Drooling	Sweating	Watery Eyes	Saliva
Motion	Cough	Hiccough, Stutter	Vocalization	Clenched Fists	Trembling
Anatomy	Nose	Mouth	Tongue	Ear	Eyes
Voice	Crying	Singing	Talking	Groaning	Shouting
Color	Pale	Yellow	Red	Dark	Gray/Green
Odor	Fishy	Fragrant	Burning	Putrifying	Oily, Greasy
Emotion	Melancholy	Anxiety, worry	Excitability	Fear	Anger

Body

Imbalances in daily life create the minor troubles that bother so many people. These imbalances produce small symptoms and can, if left untreated, develop into major problems. The body is constantly making adjustments to both the external environment and the internal environment. Many symptoms are results of this adjustment.

Problems such as fatigue, poor circulation, or depression are examples of body wide problems developing. These are the first signs that something is going wrong. The body's discharging activities are further notice of adjustment going on. The following examples point out this process. As excess has accumulated the body begins to throw off what it doesn't need. Coughing, belching, eyes tearing easy, hiccoughs, runny nose, nosebleeds, excessive ear wax, frequent urination, excessive sweating and strong body odor, diarrhea or constipation, and excessive or painful menstrual flow are some of the common symptoms that indicate the body is beginning to have trouble. The internal excesses are being discharged through the surface.

Surface body features such as skin, hair, and fingernails reflect your condition. If they are in an abnormal state this reflects the internal situation. Hair that falls out easily or that is oily, dry, or has split ends indicates overeating, especially animal and dairy foods. Skin that is abnormally colored, oily, excessively moist, dry, or prematurely wrinkled indicates problems within. If the fingernails are cracked, break easily, or have pit marks or discolorations, there is trouble with the circulation and some of the internal organs. All body features inform us of our present condition.

There are many problems that affect the body which are not quite illnesses, such as fatigue. There can also be more specific problems such as epilepsy or sciatica. The combination of shiatsu, diet, breathing, and exercise can improve both general or specific types of conditions.

Typical common problems are discussed in this chapter. For this entire group of problems, the basic full body shiatsu treatment is effective. We must remember always to consider the whole body, even when we are dealing with a specific illness. An illness rarely affects only one part of the body. Our method is to create balance without adding negative side effects.

---

fatigue

Full body shiatsu is most effective in treating fatigue. If you are short on time, you can press the bottom of the foot in the middle at acupoint KD 1. Press with a spiral movement for up to one minute. Press both feet.

After a warm shower follow with a short cold shower. This will increase vitality as it produces an alkaline condition in the blood. Deep breathing dispels CO_2 thereby leaving the body alkaline.

Moxibustion

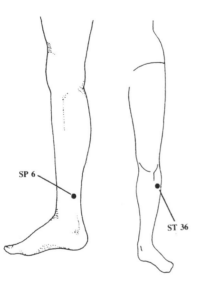

Apply moxa to acupoints ST 36, SP 6, and CV 6. Heat each point for three to five minutes, everyday or every other day until normal energy returns. Tests have shown that stimulation of these points will increase both red and white blood cell count. The red blood cells reach their peak three days after the first treatment.

Special Drinks

Twig tea with tamari. Place 1/2-1 teaspoon of tamari or good quality soy sauce into a hot cup of twig tea. This beverage creates an alkaline condition in the blood and alleviates fatigue.

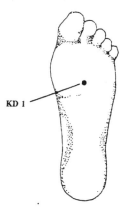

KD 1

Kuzu Drink. Dissolve a heaping teaspoon of kuzu powder into one cup of cold water. Bring the mixture to a boil, reduce the heat and stir until the liquid becomes thick and transparent. Add 1/2-1 teaspoon tamari or soy sauce and drink while hot.

When digestive trouble accompanies fatigue you can add 1/2-1 umeboshi (salted plum).

---

circulation problems
cold hands and feet
hot and sweaty hands and feet
aftereffects of stroke

Full body shiatsu can be used for all these conditions. Additionally a brisk body rub with a wet towel (either hot or cold whichever temperature that you prefer), loofa sponge or natural fiber brush will enhance circulation. It also provide an avenue for toxic material within the blood and lymph fluid to leave the body.

Cold hands and feet—use ginger hand and foot baths, alternating first hot and then cold.

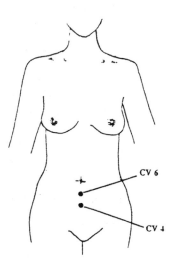

CV 6

CV 4

Sweaty hands and feet—avoid sugar, dairy, fruit juices.

Stroke and all circulation problems—avoid dairy and all fatty foods. Include shiitake mushrooms, daikon radish, or turnip. Exercise whenever possible as your condition permits. Use ginger foot bath.

---

common cold

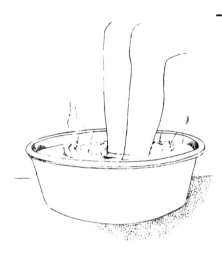

One of the most frequent illnesses is the common cold. Contrary to popular belief, cold weather does not actually appear to cause them. Studies with volunteers in the Arctic and those exposed to cold weather have not shown any increase in the number of colds. They tend to come in waves; in the U.S., the first outbreak is usually in the autumn a few weeks after schools have opened. The second wave occurs in midwinter and the third wave is in the spring.

Research has revealed that any one of over a hundred different viruses are present when someone has a cold. The illness itself is a viral infection of the upper respiratory passages.

The frequency of colds is staggering. Pre-school children have an average of six to twelve per year. Parents with small children get about six per year; other adults usually get only two to three. Half of all Americans will get a cold during the winter season.

Symptoms of colds vary with the individual. Usually there is the feeling of being ill along with sneezing and headache. This is followed by feeling chilled, a sore throat, and heavy nasal discharge. A thin, clear nasal discharge turns into a thick, yellow-green one with time. The cold can last from one to two weeks.

Because colds are so short-term and the immune system deals with them naturally, they are considered a non-medical problem. Home self-treatment is effective in lessening symptoms, as well as strengthening the body's defenses to minimize or prevent colds in the future. Having excessive mucus in the lungs and breathing passages encourages the spread of the viruses that are present with colds. Dairy foods, beef and other fatty foods, sugar, and fruit juices create excessive mucus in the body. This serves as a breeding ground for the viruses to multiply and spread. It is the fight between your body's defenses and the virus that creates the fever and other symptoms that we associate with a cold. The goal of treatment is not only to eliminate symptoms, but to strengthen the defenses so as to avoid future colds.

Shiatsu

The full body treatment serves as a preventive measure for a colds. Once one is present emphasize treatment on the back and the neck/head area.

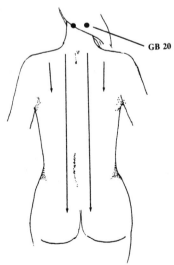

GB 20

Have the receiver lie face down. Standing astride the person, beginning at the level of the shoulder near the spine, lean your body weight into each point holding for three to five seconds. Move your thumbs down the spine toward the waist about two inches at a time. Do shiatsu on the entire area from the shoulder down to the waist. This is the urinary bladder channel. Within this area are found the referral points to all the

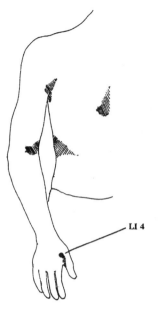

internal organs. The area between the shoulder blades may be sore, as this is the lung area. Work this area well to relieve congestion in the breathing passages and the lungs.

After completing the back, have the receiver sit in a chair or sit up on the floor. The giver places one hand on the forehead and the other at the back of the neck, and, with the thumb, press the lines on the sides of the neck. Directly under the skull are two places (GB 20)—one on each side of the neck—that are very good for relieving the cold's symptoms. In the Orient one does not catch a cold, one "catches wind." It is said that the wind resides in GB 20, "the wind pond." Stimulation of this point can disperse the wind or cold from the body.

On the front of the face, press points around the eyes, nose, and forehead. Hold each point with the thumb for several seconds making spiral motions. To clear the sinus, acupoint LI 20, "welcome fragrance," is good.

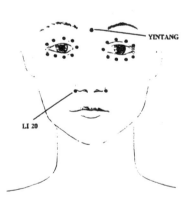

Finally, manipulating the entire hand is good to increase circulation to the lungs and upper body. Especially press acupoint LI 4 for headaches.

Diet

The overconsumption of foods like cold drinks, fruit, ice cream, sugar, and fatty foods like beef, cheese etc., contribute to the symptoms of a cold. The standard macrobiotic diet will help to prevent frequent colds.

Warm foods are especially good when a cold is present. A daily cup or two of fresh miso soup (see appendix) with a small portion of seaweed helps to strengthen the blood and tastes delicious. If the appetite is not so strong, then eat only soup. However if you have an appetite, then include whole grains and cooked beans and vegetables.

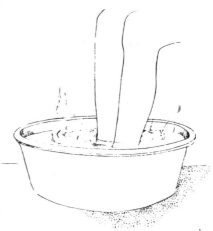

Moxibustion

Moxa on leg point ST 36 stimulates the immune system. Warm each leg for ten minutes using the bird-pecking style.

Foot Bath

Soaking the feet in a hot ginger foot bath before bed increases circulation and warms the entire body. It encourages restful sleep during which your body can heal itself.

---

arthritis pain

shoulder pain

bursitis

tennis elbow

pain and tightness between the shoulder blades

swelling (edema)

Injury to a joint, such as the elbow or shoulder, or arthritic inflammation can be quite painful. A combination of diet and shiatsu effectively deals with these common problems.

If an injury has occurred, shiatsu can inhibit swelling. It can also reduce the pain.

In the case of arthritis, the macrobiotic diet is the key in alleviating the symptoms. Extremes of food aggravate arthritic symptoms. Beef, eggs and other animal foods, fruits, fruit juice (especially tropical varieties), spices, stimulant and aromatic herbs, soft drinks, sugar, honey, chocolate, vinegar, and especially the entire nightshade family (tomato, potato, eggplant, bell pepper, and tobacco) have been linked with increased arthritic pain. In addition, oil and fat contribute to arthritis. Its symptoms are also aggravated by excessive intake of liquid and icy drinks such as soda and beer. Because of its dairy base, high sugar content, and frozen nature, ice cream is also a major exacerbating factor.

Shiatsu is also helpful in the case of arthritis., However, the diet must be followed to have lasting relief.

Diet

The standard macrobiotic diet is recommended for any joint injury and especially in the case of arthritis. Whole grains, such as millet, barley, brown rice, oats, whole wheat, rye, corn, and buckwheat should make up the majority of the diet. All vegetables should be cooked. With vegetable selection, take care to avoid tomatoes, potatoes, eggplant, asparagus, spinach, chard, avocados, beets, zucchini, and mushrooms. Cooked dried daikon with miso is beneficial and can be taken regularly. As a table seasoning, scallions cooked with miso and a few drops of sesame-oil can be used. The remainder of the diet should consist of beans, seaweed, soup, and a small volume of fish and cooked fruit occasionally (perhaps once or twice per week). All food should be chewed thoroughly.

Ginger compress

In the case of arthritis, the intestines are usually hard and stagnant. A ginger compress on the abdominal area is helpful to soften the congestion there. You can also rub up and down the spine with a hot ginger towel.

Compresses can be placed directly on the affected arthritic parts such as hands and feet. Daily compresses will accelerate blood and body fluid circulation and soften up the hardened parts. Or perhaps, if a large area is affected, you can soak either the hands or feet in a ginger bath.

Shiatsu

Shiatsu can be given to whichever area of the body has the pain. You can follow the instructions for giving a full body treatment or, if time is limited, you can use your common sense and massage the individual part. Massage must be gentle enough so as not to cause unnecessary suffering. For example, if someone has arthritis of the hand, use shiatsu on the hand according to the instructions in the treatment part of this book. Remember that the aim of treatment is to alleviate the person's suffering and increase circulation. The pressure should be firm yet yielding. That is, if the pressure is too much for the receiver, then go lighter but repeat the movement more often.

In the case of shoulder or neck trouble, be sure to include rotation and movement of the affected part. This will shorten the recovery time.

For the swelling that frequently occurs after mastectomy, light shiatsu on the upper shoulder and the lower arm of the affected side will encourage reabsorption of fluid. In addition, a buckwheat plaster can be used to pull out excess water (edema). (See appendix.)

jet lag

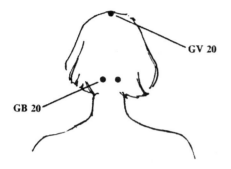

GV 20

GB 20

With the convenience of air travel, more and more people are taking advantage of flying greater distances. These long flights have a very real effect on the body. During a long flight, such as across the U.S. from one coast to the other, or a flight to Europe, the physiological functions of the body are thrown out of kilter. The body becomes imbalanced.

The body has a certain rhythm in which it operates during a twenty four hour period. This is called the "circadian" rhythm. During this cycle the body experiences slight changes of temperature, minor changes of sodium and potassium in blood levels, and changes in hormone secretions. Because of rapid time zone changes these normal functions are disrupted. How long it takes to return to normal function after a long flight depends on the individual. Some common symptoms of jet lag include: dry mouth, racing pulse, disorientation, insomnia, and often a loss of appetite.

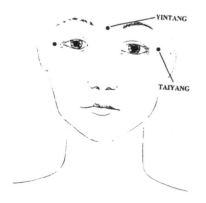

YINTANG

TAIYANG

Flights from the west to the east are more taxing. Evidence reveals that the traveler's ability to perform tasks is lower after long distance travel. It is best not to make important decisions soon after arrival.

To minimize the effects of jet lag while on the airplane, avoid alcoholic drinks, as these, along with a pressurized cabin, dehydrate you; sleep or rest as much as possible. Also try to sleep at the end of the journey rather that doing a lot of work immediately.

Shiatsu

Full body shiatsu relieves the stress of travel better then anything else. Especially press the acupoints on the neck, shoulders, and head, GB 20 and GV 20, Yintang and Taiyang.

Diet

Eat simply and be rested before the flight. Order non-dairy vegetarian meals when you make reservations for your trip. And for your stomach's sake, bring brown rice balls or sushi on the airplane with you. Brown rice is satisfying and allows you to remain feeling light rather then stuffed. With some airlines it is best to avoid the meals altogether.

After arrival at your destination, the rule of eating simply should be adhered to for at least one day.

---

numbness

paralysis

hemiplegia

paraplegia

Paralysis is the loss of muscular function in a part of the body, caused by damage to the muscles themselves or to a part of the nervous system. There are many diseases that cause these symptoms, including muscular dystrophy, myasthenia gravis, diabetes, poliomyletis, and multiple sclerosis. The most common cause is stroke, which is caused by a hemorrhage (bleeding) or blood clot in the brain.

Hemiplegia is paralysis of one side of the body resulting from damage to or disease of the part of the brain that controls the motor nervous system. The left side of the brain controls the right side of the body, and the right side of the brain controls the left side of the body. Stroke is the most common cause of this disease. After a stroke, the limbs are, at first, limp, but they soon become stiff and may suffer cramps.

Paraplegia is paralysis of the lower limbs, often accompanied by problems controlling the rectum and the bladder.

Treatment should be directed toward increasing circulation and muscle strength. Shiatsu and exercise can be helpful.

Shiatsu

Full body shiatsu with special emphasis on the affected area is necessary. Additionally, attention should be paid to the neck, spine, and kidney areas.

With the receiver lying face down, press, near the spine, the area from the shoulders down to the end of the shoulder blade. Hold each point for 3-5 seconds. Repeat many times.

Do the same type of treatment in the area near the kidneys.

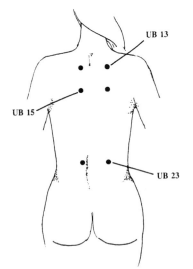

Diet

Due to the causes of stroke, either hemorrhage or blood clots, the foods which help to promote these conditions must be eliminated. These include saturated fats like those contained in meat, eggs, and dairy products, as well as sugar and other expansive (yin) foods. The standard macrobiotic diet will gradually dissolve the deposits of fat and cholesterol. Mineral rich foods like seaweeds and hard, green leafy vegetables will restore the blood vessels to their normal strength and flexibility. Oil use should also be limited, with occasional use of sesame, toasted sesame, or corn oil preferred.

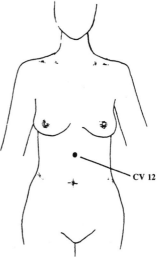

CV 12

---

epilepsy

tremor

shaking

In earlier times this illness was thought to be associated with possession by evil or even divine spirits. Actually, epilepsy is disorganized electrical activity in the brain. This leads to attacks of disturbed sensory or motor functions.

Shiatsu can be used to reduce the frequency and shorten the time of seizures. Diet is also very important. The brain and the digestive system are related.; if we can clean the intestines, then the brain will be beneficially affected.

Shiatsu

Full body treatment should be completed. Frequently pounding the head with the fist, along with deep abdominal massage is helpful.

Press GV 20, GB 20, GV 26

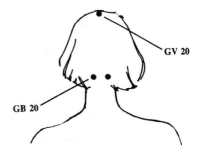

GV 20

GB 20

Moxibustion

Warm each point for 2-5 minutes.
SP 6, ST 36, UB 13, UB 15, UB 23, CV 12.

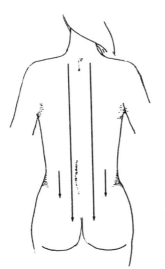

Diet

Within the standard macrobiotic diet, more strengthening foods are taken in order to control epilepsy. In addition to fifty-sixty per cent whole grains like brown rice, eat many vegetables. Also the method of cooking should incorporate a longer cooking time such as baking and a waterless style. (See macrobiotic cook books.) However for those who are very tight and rigid, their cooking should also include lightly cooked vegetables in order to soften the body.

A major cause of seizures is the repeated overconsumption of liquid. Therefore excessive drinking of water, fruit juice, milk, soft drinks, beer, wine, and alcoholic drinks should be avoided. Overeating is a common habit of people with epilepsy. Recreational activities other than eating should be encouraged.

---

overweight
big hips from overnourishment
cellulite

For cosmetic or beauty reasons, many people are concerned with their weight. Most people have good reason to be concerned. The health risks associated with an overweight condition can be serious. Illnesses such as diabetes, backache, hardening of the arteries, and osteoarthritis are the most common reasons why your doctor will recommend that you should lose weight. Most cases of obesity are caused by a calorie input that is greater than energy expenditure. In other words, people are eating more that their bodies can use. The excess is stored as fat in all the usual places around the body, the waist, hips, upper thighs, and breasts are the favorite resting places for those transformed desserts that now add unwanted girth to your once slim body. Many people are worried about the formation of cellulite which appears as dimples or lumpiness in the fatty tissue.

The way to lose weight is to reduce the calorie intake to below the body's requirements and to regulate the metabolism. The amount of food and drink put into your body must be less then the amount of energy that is used in your day to day activities. The greatest amount of weight loss usually occurs in the first week of a reducing diet, mostly because of fluid loss. A realistic weight loss goal is one to two pounds per week. Emotional factors also play a large role in eating and weight gain.

Shiatsu

Full body treatment helps to increase circulation throughout the entire body. Shiatsu also relaxes the individual so that they may gain insight into excessive eating patterns, thereby removing the emotional factors in being overweight. Remember that not everyone must look like a movie star. However, body weight should be appropriate for bone structure and your physical activity. It is certainly possible to be a few pounds over the average weight and be healthy. Superficial body fat is not the real danger. It is the fat that is stored in and around the vital 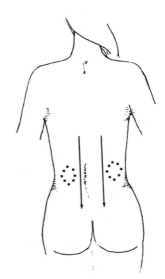 organs such as the heart that is of concern. Fat on the waist mirrors excess fat building up in vital places within.

Diet

Desserts, cream sauces, cheese, snack foods, and other high fat and high sugar foods, as well as overeating, all contribute to increased weight. It becomes clear to us that diet is the foundation for solving an overweight problem. The macrobiotic diet, which is high in complex carbohydrates (grains and vegetables) and low in refined sugars and fats is an appropriate solution. Generally, it is better to have regular, small meals than to try to starve yourself and overcompensate later with "reward" foods. Meals must be balanced and satisfying. Include a wide variety of whole grains, such as barley, corn, whole wheat, brown rice, millet, fresh garden vegetables and seaweed with miso or tamari broth soup. Avoid peanut and other nut butters as well as nuts in general. To effect the greatest weight loss, fruit intake should be limited, perhaps not even every day. Enjoying food and not suffering emotionally is the key to understanding food and putting it in its place. Food is an enjoyable part of life that allows us to live. Be honest with yourself in your relationship to it and it won't control you.

Making minor changes in the daily routine occasionally is helpful to keep your interest renewed. Changes in your exercise routine or diet go a long way to keep you interested in life and not become bored. As an example you may want to avoid salt for one week or not eat rice for three days—any change that gives you a break from the normal routine and gives you the opportunity to self-reflect. Some people enjoy fasting once a year or eating only whole grains for several days occasionally. All of these suggestions are simple yet quite helpful.

Exercise

Increase your energy output with the help of exercise. Exercise that makes the pulse increase and body sweat for twenty minutes at a time quickly burns away the pounds. Walking, swimming, dancing or aerobics can be used. Do something that you really enjoy!

---

curvature of the spine

Shiatsu on the back may relieve the pain brought on by curvature. In some cases, the curve may be slowly corrected.

Shiatsu

Have the receiver lie face down. With the giver standing directly over the receiver with one leg on each side of the body, press the back points using body weight. Lean into each point, bending the knees. Beginning at the shoulder level, work down, pressing 11/2 inches from the spine. Hold each point for 3-5 seconds. Repeat many times, spending time where hardness or pain is located.

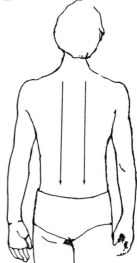

Moxibustion

Moxa heat can be applied on any hard or painful spot that you find while doing shiatsu. Do bird-pecking technique for five minutes on each point.

Ginger compress/Ginger oil

A ginger compress can be applied directly to the area of the back where the curve is the most obvious or to the area of pain. The compress will increase circulation and begin to loosen and relax the muscles that hold the spine in its curved position.

A mixture of ginger oil can be vigorously rubbed all over the back near the spine daily. This soothes and softens the muscles. (See appendix)

lumbago
back pain - strain and sprain
muscle spasm
sciatica
hip pain
imbalanced/tilted hip

It seems that almost everyone at one time or another has had some trouble with back pain. Pain in the back may be caused by muscular strain, a slipped intervertebral disk, or it may be caused by some disease of the bones and joints of the spine.

The hips are the foundation upon which rests the upper skeletal system. From the triangular center part of the pelvis, we find the twenty four vertebrae that make up the spinal column which reaches up to the skull. The spinal column consists of seven cervical, twelve thoracic and five lumbar vertebrae. These are separated by cushions of tough elastic cartilage called disks. The disks act as shock absorbers and give the back its flexibility. There are ligaments and muscles which hold the vertebrae in place. Two important muscle groups are found on each side of the spine. Within the spinal column are the spinal nerves of the central nervous system.

More often than not, backache is cause by strain of the muscles around the lower part of the spine. Doing some activity or sport that you are not used to will strain the muscles of the back. If the spine is kept erect it is less likely to have backache. Chairs that force the back to sit in a curved posture can cause chronic back strain, so TV watchers beware! Watching sports on TV can promote backache the same as playing the sport.

The pain of lumbago is often localized to one extremely painful spot in the muscles, usually in the lower lumbar region and slightly to one side of the midline. Lumbago often occurs after a combination of new exercise and cold, such as a new jogging routine in the winter or digging a garden in the spring. The spasm of the muscle fibers can be so severe that some people cannot get out of bed.

Another common cause of sudden backache is damage to one of the disks in the lower region of the spine. Lifting something heavy while the back is curved puts pressure on the disk. If enough stress is placed on the disk it will rupture and move from its normal location. The part that moves can press on the spinal nerves. Frequently, this pressure causes pain extending down the main sciatic nerve which runs from the buttock to the foot. The pain is made worse by coughing, straining, or bending the back.

Treatment for slipped or prolapsed disk is rest, with the individual flat on the back in bed. Rest for two weeks, sometimes more, often allows the protrusion to be reabsorbed back into the disk and the damaged part to heal.

Ginger compress

Place compresses directly on the back area that is in pain, alternate hot towels for at least twenty minutes. For severe backache you can do ginger compresses several times each day. Always follow the compress with shiatsu.

Shiatsu

Have the receiver lie face down, trying to relax the back muscles as much as possible. A ginger compress before the shiatsu makes the treatment more effective.

With the fingertips, probe and find the most painful area. After discovering the center of trouble, with the heel of your hand, massage lightly the sore spot in a circular direction. This will increase circulation. Then with the thumbs press with your body

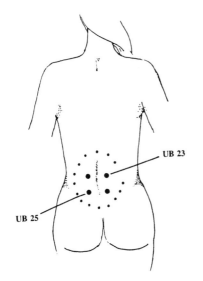

weight (standing over the person with one leg on each side) into the two muscle bands that run down the sides of the spine. These muscles have the Urinary Bladder Channel passing through them. At the level of the pelvis, lumbar 4, press especially well (UB 25). Lean your whole body into the points bending your knees and letting gravity do the work. Continue shiatsu on this area for 5-10 minutes.

After finishing the back area, you can massage several places on the backs of the legs. First, with the hands, press the upper thighs. Then with the thumbs, press down the center of the upper leg holding each point for 2-5 seconds. Press the center of the back of the knee. This is an ancient acupoint (UB 54) noted in the classics to relieve all types of back pain.

The lower part of the leg should also receive shiatsu. With the thumbs, press down rapidly in a circular motion at the center of the calf. The giver is sitting at the receiver's feet facing the head. Finish with firm pressure on the center of the calf (UB 57) and the inside and outside of the heel of the foot (UB 60 and KD 3). Pressing the bottom of the foot with the thumb is useful.

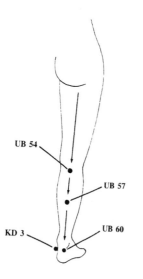

Moxibustion

The heat of moxibustion is very effective in relaxing muscles which are contracted or spasming. Apply moxa for 3-5 minutes on the following points: UB 23, UB 25, UB 57.

Exercise

A variety of exercises can be done to strengthen the lower back. They can be done either alone or with a partner. The following are just some examples of what you can do.

Leg and Head Lift

Lie face down and have both arms behind the back. Raise the legs and the upper body at the same time, stretching them backward so that a bow position is assumed. Hold for as long as possible. Rest, then repeat.

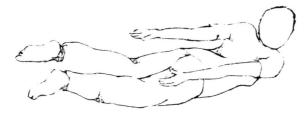

Waist Bend

Stand with feet shoulders' width apart. Bend forward at the waist and gradually move toward the floor. Bounce gently until the hands touch the floor. Then return to a standing position and bend backward at the waist. Repeat this several times. It is best if you gently push yourself with the understanding that progress is slow but sure.

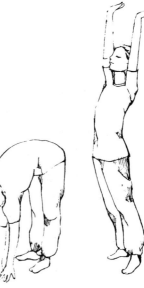

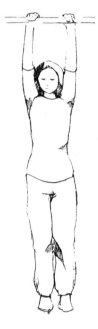

Hanging

With your hands, hang on to a bar or door frame above your head. This will stretch the spine. While hanging swing the hips forward and backward, side to side. This will rotate the lumbar area. Continue until you get tired. Then let go, rest, and repeat a few times.

Leg to Chest Lift

Lay on the back, lift and bring one knee to the chest then, back out straight again. Alternate with each leg. Do the right leg first, then follow with the left. Repeat with each leg twenty times.

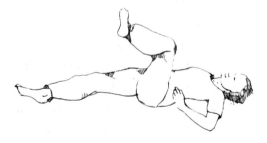

There are numerous other exercises which can be extremely useful in mending an ailing back. These exercises will also lessen the possibilities of re-injury if they are performed on a regular basis.

More important for your recovery is the fact that you can invent your own set of exercises quite easily. Examples such as standing with your arms swinging from side-to-side as you twist and look over your shoulder or gently rolling on a padded floor on your back with your hands grasping your feet. Both can loosen stiff muscles as it increases a better blood supply to the area of pain. The point is for you to develop what your body needs. As little as 5-10 minutes invested each day will pay big dividends. The alternatives to healthy home back care are medications and often times surgery. These options should not be decided upon lightly.

More classical exercise routines such as yoga, Do-In, Chinese, Korean, and Tibetan exercise programs are beneficial.

Neck

stiff neck

stiff shoulder

tightness of the neck and shoulders caused by draft

crick in the neck

whiplash

The neck is the bridge or channel between the head and body. Many important nerves and blood vessels gather in this area. If the neck is troubled, it is easy for many head problems to develop such as brain tumor, ringing in the ears, sinus congestion, headache, and glaucoma. Once established, head problems are difficult to cure. It will take a long time to change, so be persistent in the application of shiatsu.

All of the above mentioned conditions indicate varying degrees of restriction in the neck region. All neck conditions except sore throat can be treated in the same way.

Ginger Compress

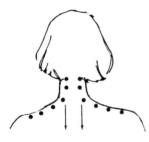

If movement is severely restricted and painful, first apply hot ginger compresses on the painful area. Approximately fifteen minutes of compresses should warm and relax the tightened area, making the effects of shiatsu much more penetrating.

Shiatsu

Knead Shoulders. The receiver is seated on the floor or in a chair while the practitioner stands behind. First, a kneading method is used to loosen up the whole shoulder and neck area. This is applied across the top of the shoulders and to the sides of the neck. This will make the person feel more comfortable and relaxed.

Press Shoulders. With the thumbs on the back of the shoulders and the other fingers laying over the top of the shoulders, press and hold with the thumbs for about five seconds. Begin near the spine and work outwards, moving every 1-1 1/2 inches toward the edge of the shoulder. There are about four to five spaces where you can hold. Repeat this several times until the muscles of the shoulders begin to soften.

Press Neck. Next, the practitioner should move from behind to beside the receiver. Place your closest hand on the back of the neck at shoulder level and the other hand on the forehead to stabilize and support the head. Your thumb is on the side of the neck closest to you and the other four fingers are on the opposite side of the neck, giving support. Hold and press with the thumb, beginning near the lower part of the ear and continuing until you reach the shoulder.

Either press and move your thumb quickly from one point to the next, or hold each point for a few seconds, depending on the pain response of the receiver. Repeat this method until the muscles become softer. You can press on three lines from the lower ear to the shoulder. Be especially attentive to the sore and painful areas. Gently making a circular press with the thumb on the painful area will increase circulation and relieve pain.

Rotate Head. Maintaining the same body position, that is, standing to the side of the receiver with one hand on the neck and the other on the forehead, rotate the neck. The range of movement should be small at first. Just guide the head first in one direction several times, then in the opposite direction several more times. While turning the neck, ask the receiver to relax the neck muscles.

Avoid producing any unnecessary pain.

Relax Muscles. Finish the treatment with chopping movements, with the sides of the hands on the area near the spine at the shoulder level and between the shoulder blades.

Neck Exercises

Stretching exercises are an important part of treatment to relieve discomfort in your neck. They help restore motion and relieve pain associated with stiffness. These exercises are more effective when performed in the shower, after a shower or following the application of hot, moist towels. Moist heat relieves pain by increasing blood flow to the muscles of your neck.

Gradually increase the number of times you repeat each exercise as your condition improves, but stop when fatigued. In the beginning five times per day may be enough, as you continue ten to twenty times per day will not be too many. They may be done intermittently during the day to help relax and relieve tension of the neck and shoulder muscles. Take an exercise break during your work day.

1. Stand erect. Turn your head slowly to the right as far as is possible without straining. Return to normal center position and relax. Repeat on other side.

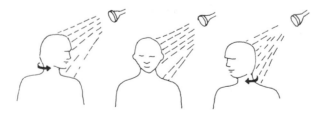

2. Stand erect. Try to touch the left ear to the left shoulder. Never force or strain. Return to normal center position and relax. Try to touch the right ear to the right shoulder. Return to normal center position and relax.

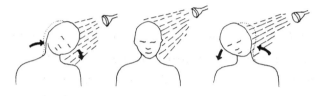

3. Stand erect. Raise both shoulders as close to the ears as possible and hold as you count to five. Relax. Stretch you shoulders backwards as far as possible and hold, then relax.

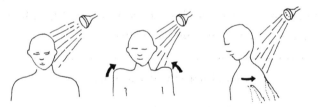

4. Stand erect. Slowly try to touch your chin to your chest. Rotate your head backwards slowly, looking up at the ceiling.

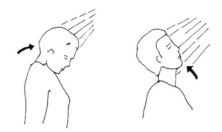

5. Stand erect. With one hand, grasp the other hand behind the back, then pull downwards towards the floor. Take a deep breath, stand on your tiptoes, and look at the ceiling while exerting the downward pull. Hold momentarily, then exhale slowly and relax. Repeat ten times.

6. Lie on your stomach with your hands clasped behind your back. Pull your shoulders back and down by pushing your hands towards your feet, pushing the shoulder blades together, and lift head from floor. Take a deep breath. Hold for two seconds. Relax.

7. Lie on back, knees flexed. Take a deep breath slowly, using elbows for support, fully expanding chest, touching top of head on the floor, then exhale slowly. Repeat ten times.

---

calcification of the neck

Avoid all dairy products including milk, cheese, ice cream, yogurt, kefir, cottage cheese, cream, butter, and cream cheese. Also avoid beef, chicken, eggs, and sugar.

Try the macrobiotic diet with the addition of seaweed and daikon radish or turnip every day.

Ginger compresses are important to loosen up the neck and

improve circulation. Repeat every night for five days. Rest for the weekend. Repeat this series until pain decreases.

---

sore throat

Do the same shiatsu treatment as described for the neck. Add acupoint LI 4 on the hands. Press point LU 11 near the base of the thumbnail with a chopstick for 5 seconds, 5-10 times. Do this on both hands. Repeat several times throughout the day.

A hot foot bath can be taken until the feet become really red. Vigorously massage and press the bottom of the foot near the base of the big toe in the arch. You will find a sore spot there. Massage this spot until it becomes less painful.

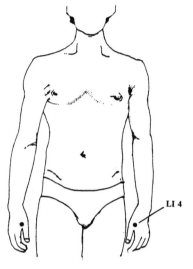

LI 4

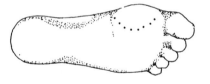

Gargle

Prepare a warm, salty solution by adding 1/2 teaspoon of sea salt to one cup warm water or twig tea. Gargle by placing a small amount of this solution in the mouth and sticking the tongue out while gargling. Repeat this several times throughout the day.

Avoid honey, sugars, spices such as chili peppers and sauces, curry, white and black pepper, and all yin food or drink.

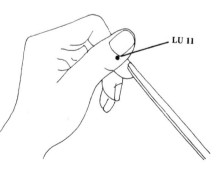

LU 11

Yoga

Try the lion's pose. Sit on the heels with the knees open or closed. You can sit on a chair if necessary. Place your hands on your knees. Open chest, look up, inhale and strongly exhale as you stick your tongue out. Stiffen the fingers and spread them wide. At the same time open both mouth and eyes wide, tensing the neck and throat. Let the feeling of tension permeate your whole body. Hold this posture for a few seconds, then relax. Repeat this several times.

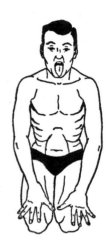

Head

headache

migraine

Headache is a very common ailment. Associated with many illnesses, it occurs without specific cause as well. Most headaches arise in tissues outside the skull. Headache is only a symptom. It can occur with the common cold, flu, sinus trouble, toothache, allergies, hay fever and other nose and eye diseases, and menstrual irregularities, to name a few. There are several kinds of headache which can be classified according to location of pain and accompanying symptoms.

One type of headache is generally found in the front part of the forehead and is of an acute nature, that is, it comes on quickly and occurs with other symptoms such as runny or stuffy nose and swollen eyes.

Another type of headache is migraine. It arises from irregular changes (dilation and constriction) in blood vessels in the scalp, temple, and face. It is usually one-sided, sudden, and very intense. Many times visual disturbances such as blank spaces before the eyes and blurred vision are present. Dizziness, nausea, and other weakening symptoms can also be present.

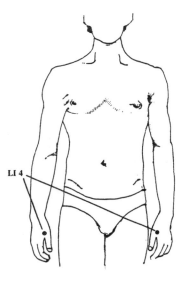

A third type is the tension headache, which is caused by stress. It is often accompanied by stiffness throughout the body. It occurs in the temples or at the back of the head or neck.

LI 4

Many simple home treatments are

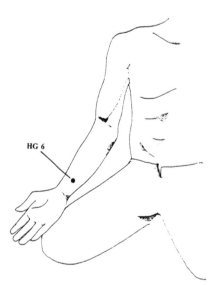

effective for headache. If you have time, a full body shiatsu is helpful to relax and calm the receiver. The full treatment will also stimulate and balance all the internal organs and is effective for all three types of headaches.

As we work to alleviate the pain of headache, we must, at the same time, be attentive to the cause. Many times the source of pain can be traced back to diet. Expansive foods such as spices, coffee, sugar, chemicals in foods (e.g., monosodium glutamate or MSG), fruit juices, fruit, soft drinks, ice cream, and other junk foods can cause dilation in the blood vessels and therefore pain. Contractive foods such as beef and all red meats, eggs, cheese, chicken, too much fish and seafood, salt, and snack foods can cause the blood vessels in the scalp, temple, and face to constrict, thereby creating pain in these areas. Many people with chronic headache eat a variety of both types of foods. A simple rule of thumb is: if you get a headache after eating expansive foods (yin), then apply a cold compress on the painful area (yang effect). If you get a headache after eating contractive foods (yang), then apply a hot compress (yin effect) where it hurts.

Palm Healing

Place one hand on the forehead and the other hand at the base of the neck. Ask the receiver to close the eyes. Have the receiver breathe in and out slowly and deeply. The giver breathes simultaneously in the same rhythm. Do this holding technique for several minutes.

Pounding

You can gently pound the top of the head with your fist many times. Also pound at the hairline. This causes contraction and is effective for expansive headaches.

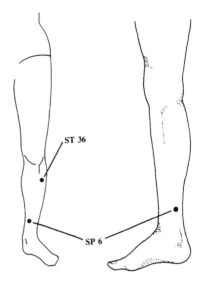

Scarf

Tightly tie a scarf or headband around the head. This contracts the head vessels and is effective for headache.

Shiatsu

Give head, shoulder, and upper-back shiatsu, and manipulate the part of the head where there is pain. First lightly pound the head with the fist. Always press the neck, shoulder, and especially the cervical region that part of the spine below the head, down to the shoulders. One hand is placed on the forehead for stability and the other is placed directly on the neck. The thumb presses from below the ear to the shoulder. Repeat this several times. Do both sides of the neck by changing your body position and your hands.

With a strong grip, knead the shoulder muscles between your thumb and forefingers, pinching slightly. Then press with the thumbs across the top of the shoulders.

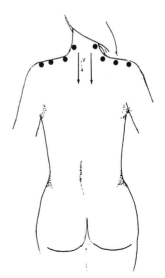

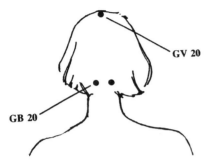

GV 20

GB 20

Other points for pressure depend on the location of the pain. In the case of front headache pain, press the points on the forehead. For pain around the eyes, press the points in that area. For temple pain, use the points in the temple beginning near the corner of the eye and moving back toward the ear. For back of the head pain, press firmly in that area.

With the thumb, press lightly over the whole head. Then press along the midline of the head, going from the front to the back, that is from the hair line toward the back. Especially press GV 20, the midpoint on the head. Any sore or tender spots are to be pressed lightly at first, then with more pressure as the receiver can tolerate it. Go back and forth over the top of the head many times.

To heighten the effect of shiatsu, press the point in the hand (LI4) which affects any problem in the head. Strongly manipulate this point for 30 seconds, at least twice on both hands or until the headache subsides. Massage other acupoints on the arms and legs such as HG 6, ST 36, and SP6.

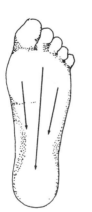

Press the sole of the foot. There is a top and bottom relationship in the body. Pressure on the bottom affects the top. Press here for several minutes.

Foot Bath

A hot foot bath brings blood circulation down to the lower parts of the body, away from the head. Soak feet for up to twenty minutes.

Walk

When you feel a headache about to come on or a mild one is already present, go for a walk in the fresh air. The air and movement will increase body circulation and eases the tension brought on by headache. Walk for a minimum of five to ten minutes.

Face

---

sinus trouble

The sinuses are cavities in the bones of the face and skull. The largest sinuses are found in the forehead and cheeks. The symptoms of pain and tenderness above them (many times with a nasal discharge) are typical signs of sinus trouble. Obstruction of normal sinus drainage by extra mucus produces the pain associated with sinusitis and stuffy nose. The affected side of the face may swell, as well as the lower eyelid.

Steam Inhalations

Stand near a kettle of boiling water and gently allow the steam to go up your sinuses. *Be careful not to burn yourself!* The steam will reduce the thickness of the mucus inside the nose and allow drainage. You should have to blow your nose after this treatment.

Ginger Compress

Ginger compresses can be placed directly on the forehead and the sinuses to loosen mucus and promote circulation. This will promote drainage. Your nose will run after the treatment. Apply for about ten minutes several times a day.

Nasal Rinse

Use one cup twig tea and 1/2 teaspoon seasalt. Liquid should be a little less salty then ocean water. Pour liquid into nasal passages and rinse. This can be done daily and is good for chronic sinusitis.

Diet

Avoid all dairy products, beef and red meats, and fried, oily or other fatty foods, such as potato chips. These increase mucus production inside the sinuses. Sugar, honey, soft drinks, and fruit juice also promote a runny nose.

Eat the standard macrobiotic diet. However, minimize breads, pancakes, and all flour products until the sinuses have cleared up. Steamed green leafy vegetables are helpful in dissolving mucus. Have at least one portion everyday. Hearty greens such as kale, cabbage, watercress, collard greens, as well as radish and turnip tops are excellent choices.

At night you can put a one-inch piece of scallion root (white part) into the nose before you go to bed and sleep with it in place. This will cause mucus drainage.

Shiatsu

Press with the fingers or rhythmically bang forehead at hairline with fist. This loosens up mucus in the frontal sinus.

Have the receiver seated, either on the floor or in a chair. Standing behind, press, with the thumbs, the area near the spine at the level of the shoulders. Press the medulla oblongata point. Massaging this area stimulates sympathetic nerves which cause contraction in the blood vessels of the nasal mucous membrane. This opens the nasal passage, allowing easier breathing.

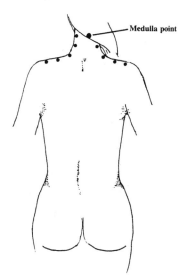
Medulla point

With the receiver lying on the back, you can press the many acupoints on the sides

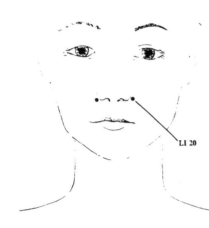

of the nose and the top of the head. Particularly good at clearing the sinuses are LI 20 ("welcome fragrance").

---

nose bleeds (epistaxis)

Many times an accidental bumping or blow to the bridge of the nose causes bleeding. This occurs because one of the fragile blood vessels in the nasal mucous membrane breaks. This minor type of problem responds quickly to treatment and is of little medical significance. Nosebleeds, however, can occur spontaneously, sometimes due to high blood pressure, nasal allergies, and/or excessive sneezing. Some people also get nose bleeds after eating certain foods such as chocolate, or drinking beverages which contain caffeine. These substances and foods high in phosphorus cause the blood vessels to expand and burst so that the nose bleeds. People who have frequent nosebleeds may have polyps—growths within the nose.

Self-Treatment

The sufferer should sit up straight with the head held forwards. While breathing through the opened mouth, grasp the soft part of the nose between the fingers and thumb to close the nostrils down onto the septum the fleshy divider between the two halves of the nose. This pressure should be held until the bleeding stops. After the bleeding stops, do not squeeze the nose again or blow it for at least forty-eight hours.

Shiatsu

The receiver should be seated. Have the receiver look up. With the side of the hand hit the back of the neck below the skull. Continue this gentle striking for a few minutes.

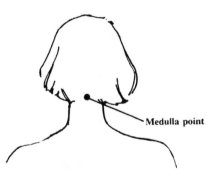

Medulla point

Then, the giver stands to the side and places one hand on the forehead to stabilize it. The other hand is placed on the back of the neck. With the thumb, treat the medulla oblongata point at the base of the skull in the center of the neck. Have the receiver breathe in a full breath as you do the same. On an exhalation, gently rock the head back onto the thumb and hold for 3 seconds. Repeat this 5-7 times. This pressure stimulates the medulla oblongata to cause constriction in the blood vessels within the nose.

---

eye fatigue

nearsightedness (Myopia)

blurred vision

eye pain

Poets throughout the ages have often looked upon the eyes as the "windows of the soul". With a somewhat less romantic view, we can see that the eyes and their surrounding tissues are among the body's most delicate structures. Most of us value our gift of sight above all other senses. The eye is actually a direct extension of the brain. The retina—the light-sensitive structure at the back of the eye—contains millions of rods and cones, which are specialized nerve endings which convert light into electrical impulses. These impulses are then conveyed by the optic nerve to the visual center at the back of the brain, where the individual interprets them as specific images.

In Oriental medicine the sense of vision and the eyes are under the control of the liver. If eye sight is failing it is the liver that is also failing in its function. The whole body with all the internal organ functions are represented in the eye. With study one can diagnose many body conditions from observation of the eyes. They represent the physical, mental, and spiritual parts of a person.

Self-Shiatsu

With the thumbs, press against the upper inside corners of the eye sockets, below the eyebrow. Then, with the thumb and index finger of one hand, squeeze the base of the nose near the corner of the eyes. First press down, then squeeze and press upward, doing first one way

With your four fingers press the upper eye rim and then the lower rim.

With the middle finger press the Yintang point, directly in the center of the two eyebrows. Hold for several seconds. With the thumbs press the temples (Taiyang points.)

Finally, apply pressure to the eyelids with the thumbs for about 10 seconds.

Shiatsu

The points and areas of treatment are much the same for partner shiatsu as for self shiatsu. When working on someone else, press the shoulders and back of the neck. This will increase circulation to the head and eye area.

---

watery eyes

This condition is caused by fruits, fruit juice, sugar, and other excessive yin substances. Place a drop or two of pure toasted sesame oil directly in the eyes with an eyedropper, preferably before sleeping. The first few applications can sometimes sting. Continue one to three days, until the eyes improve. Next morning wash with salted twig tea. Before using the sesame oil for this purpose, boil and strain with a sanitized cheesecloth to remove any impurities and let cool to room temperature.

Simple Eye Exercises

Twice a day, in almost every school in China and in many factories as well, the Chinese take a break and do four simple eye exercises, which take only ten minutes. The exercises relax the focusing muscles of the eyes and increase blood circulation.

When doing exercises, keep your eyes closed. Fingernails should be short and your hands clean. Press lightly and slowly; don't use excessive pressure. Repeat each exercise eight times, once in the morning and once in the afternoon. Sit with the elbows resting on a table.

1. Use thumbs to massage inside eyebrow corners; other fingers are slightly curled against forehead.

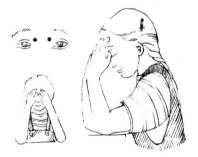

2. Use the thumb and index finger to massage the nose bridge. Press downward, then upward.

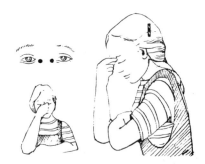

3. Place thumbs on lower jaw and index and middle fingers against both sides of nose near nostrils. Lower the middle fingers and massage with index fingers.

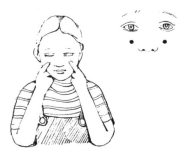

4. With fingers curled under and thumbs on each side of forehead, use the sides of the index fingers to rub outward, following the contours of the eyebrow and bony rim under the eye.

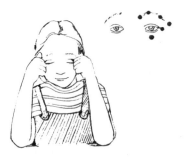

ringing in the ear (tinnitus)
ear infection
hearing loss

The ear we see attached to the side of the head is only part of the wonderful mechanism that allows us to hear the world around us. The sounds of the birds chirping, water rushing downstream, and the breeze gently moving through the trees are made possible by the interaction of sound vibrations, liquid vibrations, and electrical impulses.

These sounds enter the outer ear, that is, the structure that you and I know as our ears. These vibrations place pressure on the ear drum which is inside the middle ear. There are some small bones inside this middle portion of the ear, named the hammer, anvil, and stirrup. They conduct the vibrations from outside the ear to the ear drum and increase the intensity by seventeen times. Farther in the ear, there is the cochlea which looks like a small snail shell and acts to receive sound vibrations. Vibration continues to travel by passing through the liquid contained in the snail shell, like the movement of energy through waves in the ocean. When vibrations of the liquid in the inner ear reach another membrane (like the ear-drum), this creates a force even stronger then before. The rubbing action on some tiny hair-like cells within the inner ear makes electrical signals that travel to the brain to be translated into familiar sounds.

There are also structures in the ear that help us to maintain balance. All ear structures must work well in order for hearing to be at its best.

Many hearing and ear difficulties come from excessive ear wax, mucus, or mineral deposits, which harden and block the passages within the different parts of the ear. Treatment is aimed at

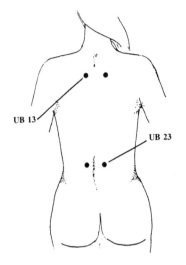

UB 13

UB 23

loosening and removing these deposits so that sound vibrations, liquid vibrations, and electrical impulses can move freely.

In traditional Chinese medicine, there is a relationship between the ears, hearing, and the kidneys. Our treatment must also strengthen both the kidneys and the circulation of energy that goes to and from the kidneys.

Shiatsu

Pull and massage the ears vigorously.

Put the index fingers into ear and wiggle fingers up and down, sending vibrations into the ear. Open mouth and move jaw back and forth to open the ear canal.

Full body shiatsu to help improve the general condition is important. During the full treatment, emphasize direct treatment of the ear as described above. In addition to the areas around the ear, the following acupoints should be pressed: UB 23, KD 3.

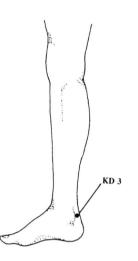

KD 3

Moxibustion

Hold the lighted moxa roll directly in front of the ear canal. With the bird-pecking motion, allow the heat to penetrate the ear for 5-10 minutes.

Salt Pack

Place a salt pack directly on the affected ear. The receiver can be lying on his or her side. Keep the salt pack on for at least fifteen minutes.

Diet

The macrobiotic diet is low in fats and oils and therefore low in foods that create excessive mucus or cause stagnation. When ear trouble is present, especially ringing in the ears, eliminate all foods which cause excessive earwax and mucus production. This includes all fried, greasy, and oily foods (including potato chips, tempura, etc,), all dairy products (especially ice cream), fruit juice, fresh fruit, and sugary items. Eliminate or at least reduce the use of flour products including breads, pancakes, and baked desserts. All of these foods create excessive earwax production as well as mucus. The use of dissolving foods such as daikon radish and turnip are useful on a daily basis.

---

stuttering

The stutterer must know that the principle cause of the condition is tension. The individual must learn to relax the upper body muscles which cause stuttering.

Shiatsu

Full body shiatsu is the best solution. Shiatsu will bring about general body-wide relaxation.

Additionally, shiatsu and moxibustion have been used successfully to relieve anxiety and relax the body. For moxibustion use: CV 12, UB 23 and UB 13.

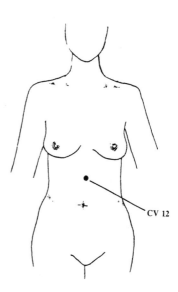

CV 12

---

toothache
impaired gum circulation
jaw dislocation

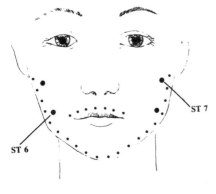

Decay of the teeth by bacteria is the primary cause of dental caries (cavities) and tooth and gum pain. Of all human diseases, dental diseases are the most common. Many people believe that loss of some or all of our permanent teeth is inevitable. This is not true if some preventive care is taken. Once some tooth or gum pain is present, you have already passed the early stage of the disease's development. Unlike other maladies where the immune system can cure the body, this is not the case with cavities. Problems can become progressively worse until proper treatment is received. This may include a dentist.

Prevention

The first important step is avoiding sticky, sweet foods upon which bacteria thrive. Sugar, candy, honey, and sticky, rich desserts are some foods that remain in the mouth, on the gums and teeth. Brushing and flossing will remove these food particles. Brushing with salted water or dentie (charred eggplant with seasalt, available in natural food stores) keeps the inside of the mouth alkaline. It is the buildup of acids, made by bacteria eating the food particles left on the teeth, that creates cavities.

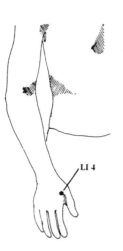

Shiatsu

Press the acupoints around the mouth and teeth. This area will improve circulation and lessen pain. For jaw dislocation was well as toothache pain, acupoints ST 6, ST 7, and LI 4 can be used successfully. You can also press the back of the jaw below the ear. Acupuncture is effective for toothache pain.

Diet

The macrobiotic diet can prevent new dental problems from arising. However, previous cavities should be cared for properly. Nutrition is directly linked to creating good strong teeth as well as to healing disorders. Proper vitamins, minerals, and food nutrients must be included in the daily diet. In addition to whole grains, beans, etc., seaweed and green leafy vegetables are important to insure that our teeth will last a lifetime.

When tooth pain is present, strictly avoid expansive foods, such as alcohol, sugar, fruit juice, etc. These will inflame the condition and increase the pain. Taking small pieces of salted plum or other salty condiments will contract the painful area. A small piece of salted plum (umeboshi) can be placed directly in the mouth on the painful area.

Dental plaque is caused by overeating, especially sweets and animal foods. Diet and cleaning the teeth are important prevention.

---

bleeding gums

Put seasalt on index finger and massage gums several times each day. Sucking on an umeboshi pit helps contract blood vessels in the gums.

Feet

---

cold feet

sole pain

heel pain

bunion pain

sprained ankle

swollen legs and ankles

slow healing after broken bones

dislocated kneecap and puffed-up knee

swollen knee

We can walk and move because of our feet, legs, and hips. When problems affect the lower part of the body, it can be extremely frustrating. Illness or injury in these areas is very common. Many people suffer from a variety of complaints, all of which limit their mobility and enjoyment of life. Shiatsu is effective in alleviating many foot, ankle, leg, and hip complaints. Once the initial pain has been relieved, regular exercise is important both for strengthening and keeping the area in use.

Treatment:

For circulatory problems in the lower half of the body such as cold feet, cramps, slow healing, varicose veins, gout, and swelling, a full body shiatsu is effective.

When specific injury causes the problem, then we must work directly on the injured part.

Soak feet in a hot ginger foot bath followed by a cold foot bath. This improves circulation to the feet.

For the heel - massage around the ankle bones, both inside and outside. After shiatsu is completed, moxibustion will further increase circulation. Warm the whole area with the moxa roll.

For the knee - when the knee is twisted and minor ligament or muscle strain occurs, ginger compress, shiatsu, and moxibustion effectively promote healing. With the receiver lying on the back, apply shiatsu above and below the knee to increase circulation to the area. Then, with the thumbs, press around the kneecap. Pay special attention to any sore spots. You can massage a mixture of 50% freshly grated ginger root juice and 50% sesame oil into the painful spots. Repeat this treatment twice each day. It takes a long time to repair the knee, so continue the treatment for one to three months and be mindful of not straining the knee further while it is healing.

---

gout

Gout is usually experienced as a sudden and extremely painful attack, most often affecting the joint of the big toe. The tissues around the joint are also inflamed in most cases, producing heat, swelling, redness, and excruciating pain and tenderness. Without treatment, more attacks can be expected. The disease results from the accumulation in the bloodstream of a waste product of metabolism known as uric acid. It is the deposit of uric acid crystals in the skin, joints, and kidneys which causes the painful symptoms. About 15-20% of gout sufferers have kidney stones which can lead to kidney failure and death.

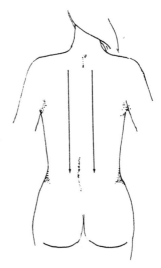

Middle-aged men are particularly affected. It is thought that their lifestyle of eating large quantities of beef and other red meat along with alcohol is directly related to gout.

Shiatsu

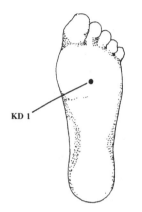

KD 1

Full body shiatsu helps to remove toxins from the blood. Additionally, attention should be directed to strengthening the kidneys. Massage the area from below the shoulder blades to the waist; repeat several times.

Also, press the bottom of the foot at acupoint KD 1 and along the inside near the arch.

Diet

Strictly avoid all meat products (including beef, chicken, lamb, pork), eggs, fish, shellfish, dairy products, sugar, spices, alcohol, honey, and other foods not normally used on the macrobiotic diet. Also avoid spinach, chard, beets, asparagus, potatoes, tomatoes, and eggplant. Use of beans should be minimal as they contain elements that can aggravate gout.

The macrobiotic diet should be adopted with plenty of fresh vegetables, including cooked leafy greens everyday. Cabbage, watercress, daikon radish tops, bok choy, etc., are good choices.

Green Compress

This compress can be placed on the painful gout area. It can reduce inflammation and pulls out excessive heat from the body.

---

clubfoot

This is a deformity present at birth which prevents the foot from being placed flat on the ground. Clubfoot affects boys twice as often as girls. It is usually found in both feet.

Shiatsu

The foot and leg part of the complete shiatsu session should be applied daily to the developing child's legs and feet. A long period of treatment is required to effect change.

Diet

The standard macrobiotic diet with an emphasis on seaweed, seeds and root vegetables supplies abundant minerals. These strengthen the muscles and bones, thus providing the support required to maintain the correct position fostered by shiatsu.

---

cramps

Cramps are caused from mineral imbalance and lack of circulation. The problem begins in the intestines. Keep the intestine clean with a high fiber diet (found in whole grains) and you shouldn't have cramps.

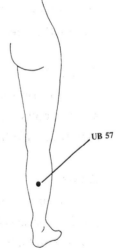

UB 57

Shiatsu

The treatment of muscle cramp is to relax the spasm and improve the local circulation. Keeping the limb warm, rubbing and massaging it, and avoiding excessive fatigue are useful in the care of cramps.

Diet

Miso soup along with seaweed supplies the minerals necessary to relieve and prevent cramps.

varicose veins

Veins contain non-return valves which allow blood to flow only toward the heart, while the veins themselves are compressed by the contraction of the muscles with each movement of the limb. In this way, blood is forced to move. When the blood passes a valve, it cannot return; more muscle contractions will then force it further up the vein.

When this valve system becomes defective, the veins of the lower part of the leg become swollen by the pressure of the column of blood in the veins higher up the leg. This swelling causes the veins to become larger and knotted. This condition is called varicose veins.

Varicose veins are a relatively common condition. They can be painless or they can cause aching, swelling, eczema, and ulceration as they become distended, enlarged, and twisted.

Seasalt Rub

Put seasalt in the palm of your wet hand. Strongly rub damp salt directly on protruding veins. After this treatment, pat the legs very well with the flat palm of the hand, then wash off saltiness.

Shiatsu

Shiatsu on the legs and feet will increase circulation and supply the compression that is necessary to force the blood in the veins to move. Full body shiatsu helps strengthen the whole body.

Exercise

Movement of any type is recommended, especially walking. Usually varicose veins are more of a problem for those who are not active.

Hot/Cold Compress

Apply a hot compress first for two minutes followed by a cold compress for a couple of minutes. Repeat the alternation of the hot/cold compresses several times ending with a cold compress.

Diet

Expansive foods such as sugar, fruit juice, chemical additives, and excessive liquids contribute to the expansion of the veins. Avoid such foods and add mineral rich foods such as seaweed, green leafy vegetables, and root crops (turnip, carrot, radish, rutabaga, burdock).

Children's Problems

Children are a precious gift. When a child gets sick it is the parents who also suffer. They often feel helpless when their offspring experience pains, aches, fever, nausea, etc. In parenting there is the feeling that one must provide food, shelter, role models, education, and healing care. When sickness occurs, being untrained or unfamiliar in the healing area can lead to fear and worry.

Parents are the major educating source for their child. The health problems that occur in adult life, such as heart disease, cancer, stroke, and accidents, are the major causes of death. Nonfatal disabilities such as arthritis, back and hip problems, and hypertension, affect a very large number of people nationwide. It is the job of the parent to teach the child how to prevent these disorders from occurring later in life. Parents themselves must be educated so that they in turn can give guidance regarding preventive measures and healthy life styles.

Abdominal pain and digestive troubles are fairly common in children from time to time. Eating too many sweet things, eating too much before bedtime, or a number of other food related activities can cause minor stomach or abdominal upset. These troubles can be opportunities for the parent to begin to discuss the effects of different foods on the child. Asking, "Why do you think your tummy hurt so much last night? Do you think it could have been the birthday cake?" begins to make the child ponder on the cause and effect of eating. This is not a time to criticize the child. It is a time to discuss without finding blame. The child already has suffered the results of his/her choice. The discussion is a chance to become aware of that fact.

Abdominal pain is more likely to be significant if it is sharply localized and constant, especially if it occurs during the night and wakens the child from sleep. Fever, vomiting, loss of appetite, or weight loss should alert you that the condition could be more than minor. If these symptoms persist and your home treatments are ineffective, you should consult with a health care professional whom you trust. Natural healing techniques can be used for the minor complaints that all children have. Usually children respond very quickly to these treatments.

---

digestive trouble

Wrong eating is almost always the cause of stomach trouble. Don't give the child sweets, including honey, fruit juice, etc. at this time. Very softly cooked brown rice or a kuzu drink (see appendix) will calm the upset stomach. Soft-cooked vegetables can also be added to the diet.

Shiatsu and/or palm healing can be done to the child. If the pain is in the stomach, press the back directly behind the stomach. You will find some tender spots there. Press them gently for about five minutes. Then, on the abdomen, rub the tummy gently and finish by placing your palm directly over the painful area and hold for a few minutes.

Ginger compress can be used.

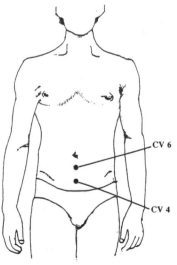

---

bedwetting (enuresis)

Drinking beverages before going to bed, emotional difficulties and generally improper eating habits (such as too many watery foods like fruit and fruit juice) all have their effect on the function of the kidney and bladder. It is best not to eat or drink two to three hours before going to bed. While many times the child will outgrow the problem, proper diet and shiatsu certainly will speed up the process. Don't scold the child.

Gentle shiatsu on the lower pelvic and sacrum areas affects the bladder. Also massage on the legs will increase the energetic flow to and from the bladder. Finally, pressing the acupoints below the navel (CV 4, CV 6) strengthens the urinary functions.

Moxibustion

Warming the following acupoints will treat the problem: CV 4, CV 6, SP 6, KD3, and LV 1

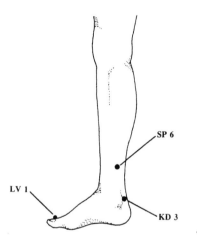

Exercise

Leg stretching exercises which stretch the inner leg and the groin can be done. The same types of exercise that is effective for prostate trouble is effective here. These can be done before bedtime. One simple exercise is to sit on the floor with the legs out at a forty-five degree angle in front. Bend forward and try to lay the chest on the floor. Repeat this up and down movement several times.

---

fever

If a slight fever is present it can be dealt with easily at home. If the fever is high and medical attention is necessary, you can also do the following until you can get to a doctor.

Sponge the child or put into a cool bath.

Mix a little apple juice with twig tea and give to the child.

Place a cabbage leaf or a tofu plaster on the child's head.

burn

Each burn case must be watched carefully. Burns from hot water, fire ,and hot oil can be treated the same. For small children don't put ice on the burn; this is too strong for them. It contracts the outside skin with the heat trapped inside. Because of this the burn can't heal quickly. Cool water or tofu plaster is appropriate.

If the burn is minor, then a little oil placed directly on the skin covered with green leafy vegetables is appropriate to use after the cool water application. Because sesame, corn, or olive oils are recommended for everyday cooking, you may have these on hand. However, any oil that you have in the kitchen will do. Cabbage, kale, dandelion, or any other available green leaf vegetable can be used for the cooling outer wrapper.

As a first aid measure, immediately put miso paste or tamari on the burn. This seals out air and stops blisters from forming. This works very well. A couple of days later, the oil and green leafy vegetable combination can be used to cover the wound. If there is swelling, tofu plaster with greens is helpful to reduce it.

For a more severe burn, don't use oil. Seek medical attention.

bruising
sprains
swollen ankles

For bruising and sprains, palm healing and light massage directly on the hurt will increase circulation, ease pain, and promote recovery. If someone bruises easily this indicates too much sugar has been eaten. Easily sprained ankles or recurring ankle sprains indicate the gall bladder may be sluggish in its function. Don't eat meat or fatty foods. Instead of eating it, use hamburger as a poultice on swollen ankles. The fat in the meat takes out inflammation and swelling—it really works! Don't touch the ankle for at least twenty-four hours. After one day's rest, administer hot and cold foot baths and shiatsu manipulation.

---

cuts

If your child cuts a finger , immediately put the finger in your mouth to cover with saliva. Raise the hand above the head and shake the hand. After doing this put miso and green leafy vegetables on the cut and bandage it.

---

emotional troubles such as frustration

Adjustments in the diet should be made so that refined sugars are not included. Regular parent/child playing, such as doing a shiatsu treatment together, will bring a sense of security to the child and a bonding with the parents. Parents can help their children by encouraging them to honestly express themselves.

Emotional and Mental Conditions

Traditional natural healing has always linked the body and mind together. It is felt that physical problems will create mental or emotional states and that prolonged negative emotions can adversely affect the internal organs. Our emotions are reflections of our mental state and are produced by various stimulations in the environment. These include one's job, relationships, and thoughts about oneself. Generally, emotions have a changing nature. They come and go. However, if the emotions are very intense and persistent or the individual is hypersensitive to the stimulations, they may result in a deep change of outlook on life and lead to disease.

The following chart shows the internal organs and the emotional and mental states connected with these organs. To effectively treat the problem, a combination of the macrobiotic diet and treating specific areas with shiatsu can be done. For example, someone suffering from depression should specifically have the lung, large intestine, and liver areas treated. (See appropriate treatment section in this book for details). Also breathing, either as an exercise or in the form of long walks, will alleviate the depressed attitude.

The aim of treatment is to remove physical rigidity thus making the body flexible. This in turn will relieve mental rigidity. If you are overly sensitive or have any mental problem, try to use your body more. Movement will make you feel more balanced.

Emotional and Mental Conditions

Area of Treatment		Conditon
Heart		Hyperactivity/Excitability
Heart		Hysteria
Liver, Lung and Large Intestine		Depression
Heart and Liver		Mental Instability
Liver and Heart		Insomnia
Liver		Anger
Liver and Gall Bladder		Irritability
Stomach		Worry
Pancreas and Spleen		Poor Memory
Pancreas and Spleen		Inability to Concentrate
Kidney		Lack of Confidence
Kidney and Stomach		Fear

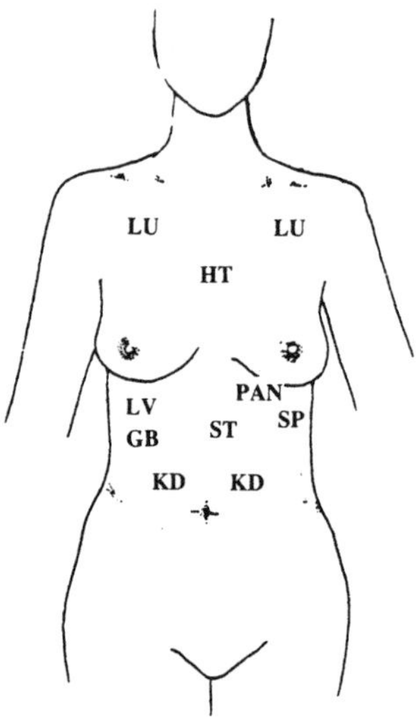

LU   LU
HT
LV   PAN   SP
GB   ST
KD   KD

To use the above chart effectively first determine which emotional state the receiver experiences most often. Match up the corresponding physical areas, located directly across from the emotions list. Treat the physical area with shiatsu and other appropriate techniques described in the respective sections found in this book. Additionally, help the receiver to understand the source of the emotional trouble through counseling and discussion. Macrobiotic and Oriental medicine see the body and mind as inseparable. "The Body and Mind are not two." This simple approach is quite effective.

First Aid

---

unconsciousness

A primary aim of first aid for someone who is unconscious is to protect the victim from choking. The individual's own tongue, along with blood, saliva, or vomit, are the things which block the windpipe and stop breathing. You can avoid the risk of suffocation by bending the person's head back and pulling his or her jaw forward. This simple movement prevents the relaxed tongue from blocking air to the windpipe. You can also put the person in the recovery position. It is safe, comfortable, and relaxing. In this position the injured person can breathe freely, and fluids such as blood or vomit can escape from the mouth, lessening the risk of choking.

Shiatsu

With the victim laying on his or her back, you can pick up the head and rotate it lightly from side to side making an adjustment. Also you can press the center of the sole of the foot (KD1) with the thumb very strongly. Pressing the acupoint (GV 26) above the center of the upper lip is helpful. These will help recover consciousness.

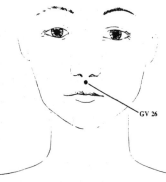

---

fainting

If the person is feeling faint, dizzy, or seasick, and is still conscious, help him or her to lie down at once. Raise the legs, loosen tight clothing, and put a cover on the person. Encourage him or her to relax and to breathe slow, deep breaths. Have the person continue to lie down until proper face color returns. Shiatsu on acupoint (GV 26) above the center of the upper lip is helpful.

If twig tea with a teaspoon of soy sauce is available, let the person drink this.

An effective self-treatment is to open the mouth, then use the thumb to strongly press the roof of the mouth while the person exhales. This immediately affects the brain.

Recovery Position

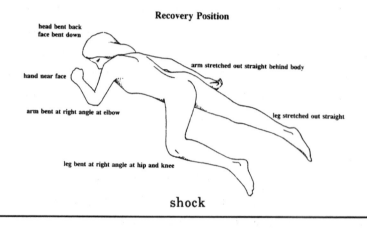

head bent back
face bent down

arm stretched out straight behind body

hand near face

arm bent at right angle at elbow

leg stretched out straight

leg bent at right angle at hip and knee

shock

Loss of blood is the cause of shock. One who has suffered injury and hemorrhages is at risk of shock. The loss of blood results in a weakened heartbeat and an inadequate supply of oxygen and other chemicals to all the tissues. It is the brain, heart, and lungs which particularly suffer. A person in shock is pale, cold, sweating, and has a fast, weak pulse. He or she also feels faint, is nauseated, and thirsty. To prevent shock lay the person on his or her side in the recovery position. Keep warm; do not provide anything to eat or drink. Alcohol can be dangerous as it can dilate the blood vessels and draw blood away from inside the body. Cigarettes are also harmful at this time as they reduce the oxygen capacity of the blood and reduce the blood supply to the heart. When the victim appears more stable, twig tea with one teaspoon of tamari soy sauce is helpful.

---

heat exhaustion

When we get hot, perspiration forms and evaporates. This pulls heat out of the body and maintains normal body temperature. The sweat also carries fair amounts of salts with it which are important for the body. A deficiency of these salts causes weakness and sometimes severe cramps.

Heat exhaustion occurs when someone has perspired heavily after long exertion or on a very hot day. The body will then lose an excessive amount of water and salts. In this condition body temperature will normally rise only slightly. The person feels faint, exhausted, and sometimes nauseated. The skin is moist and looks pale. The pulse becomes fast and feeble. Cramps may develop.

Treatment:

Get the person into a cool place and have him or her lie down. Loosen any tight clothing and raise the feet. Slightly salty drinks such as twig tea with soy sauce or water boiled with salted plums (umeboshi), are very good. Recovery should be soon.

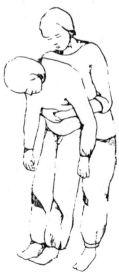

---

choking

When an individual with something lodged in the windpipe tries to dislodge it by coughing, the muscles in the windpipe tend to tighten around it and hold it.

Treatment:

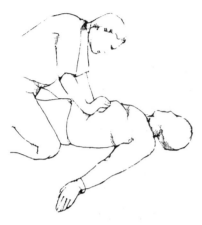

Open the person's mouth widely; with your finger feel deeply for anything at the back of the throat and pull it out. If the object is too deep for you to reach, tell the person to try to relax and to breathe deeply and very slowly. This helps to relax the spasm of the windpipe. If the object does not clear and the person is becoming blue and weak, give several hard slaps between the shoulder blades. A very small child can be held upside down by the ankles with one hand, and the other hand can slap the back.

If the person is unconscious and limp, give mouth-to-mouth artificial respiration. This relaxes the windpipe spasm and your air can pass around the object without danger of pushing it further down.

An abdominal thrust for choking can be done when food is swallowed and totally blocks the windpipe. Wrap your arms around the waist from behind. Put one fist with its thumb edge on the upper abdomen, your other hand clutching the fist. Thrust hard, inward, and upward.

If the person is lying down, place him or her quickly on the back. Kneel astride the hips. Thrust with the heel of one hand covered by the other hand in the edge of the upper abdomen—the pit of the stomach.

If a small sized object or food is stuck in the throat, it may be able to be swallowed by giving a mouthful of cooked brown rice. This will cover the object and push it down.

APPENDIX

Home Remedies

The following home remedies have been mentioned throughout this book to be used together with other treatments, such as shiatsu, exercise, and so forth. They are simple to apply. Most of the materials needed are generally available in markets and natural food stores.

Buckwheat Plaster

The buckwheat plaster is used to draw out any swelling on the body. This plaster can be applied anywhere on the body. It is commonly used on a swollen abdomen or swollen joints.

Mix buckwheat flour with enough hot water to form a hard, stiff dough. Apply in a 1/2 inch layer to the affected area. Tie in place with a cotton cloth and leave for up to four hours. The plaster itself may become watery from the fluids that created the swelling. The plaster will usually eliminate the swelling after a few applications. However, it can take up to two-three days.

Douche

Douching is unnecessary for women with normal vaginal secretions. Generally, pregnant women should not douche. In the case of any vaginal irritation, it may be useful to wash out the vagina with a cleansing stream of water or douche solution. Allow 5-10 minutes for the treatment.

For ordinary infections such as vaginitis and cervicitis, a series of treatments consists of three douches daily for three days. Then, two douches daily for three days, and once daily for thirty days. For pregnant women, a hot foot bath can be safely taken instead of a douche.

A simple douche can be made from: 7 cups water or twig tea, 2-3 inch piece of kombu seaweed, 3-4 salted plums or 1 teaspoon sea salt. Mix all ingredients together and simmer for ten minutes, strain and allow to cool. Use this liquid for douche.

Ginger Compress

This compress can relax muscle tension and promote circulation of body fluids such as blood and lymph fluid. It has a stimulation effect and helps to reduce stagnation.

Bring three to four quarts of water to boil, place about a golf ball size of fresh grated ginger root in a cotton cloth, cheesecloth or a handkerchief. Put this ball into the boiled water which is now just below the boiling point. Don't let the liquid boil again as this lessens its effectiveness. The mixture is now ready to use. Dip a towel into the hot ginger water trying to keep the ends dry, as the liquid is very hot. Hold by the ends of the towel and dip in the center portion. Wring it out and place directly on the area to be treated. Place a second, dry towel on top to reduce heat loss. Apply a fresh hot towel every minute or so and continue until the skin becomes red, about 15- 20 minutes.

Ginger Oil

The combination of fifty percent fresh ginger root juice and fifty percent good quality sesame oil when vigorously rubbed on the skin will soothe and soften muscles.

Green Compress

The green compress can draw heat out of the body. It can be used on inflamed areas. Mash up two-three leaves of cabbage greens or other available green leafy vegetable, and place directly on affected area. When leaves are warm, replace with fresh compress.

Hip Bath

This bath helps to stimulate circulation and to treat various disorders of the skin and female sex organs. Save your daikon greens and dry them in the shade away from direct sunlight. Turnip greens can be used as a substitute. Boil four bunches of dried greens in four quarts of water until the water turns brown. Add a handful of seasalt and put this liquid into the bathtub. The bath water should be at least waist high and as hot as you can tolerate. Cover the upper portion of the body with a towel. This will cause sweating. This bath is best done at night so that you can go to bed and rest afterwards. It can be repeated as needed up to ten days. If you like, you can follow the hip bath with a *douche*.

Miso Soup

Miso soup is a strengthener for the whole body. After eating miso soup you always feel much better. Scientists have discovered that properties in miso help the body to rid itself of harmful material such as pollution and radioactive particles. It has enzymes, positive bacteria which aid digestion, iron and it makes the blood alkaline. Its protein content is substantial as well.

> 2 cups water
>
> 3 inch piece wakame seaweed
>
> 1/2 onion
>
> 1/2-1 1/2 tablespoons barley miso (organic and
> unpasteurized)

Cut wakame into small pieces and place in pot and bring to boil. Cut onion and add to pot. After about 3-4 minutes the vegetables are ready. Dilute miso in a little of the soup liquid and add back to the pot. Let simmer for 2-3 minutes.

This is a basic miso soup. You can add as many other vegetables as you like. Be creative.

Salt Pack

The salt pack can be used to warm any part of the body. Roast salt in a dry pan until hot and then wrap in a thick cotton linen or towel. Apply to the troubled area and change when the pack begins to cool.

Shiitake Mushroom Tea

This tea is used to relax the body. It can also help to dissolve accumulated animal fats, stored in the body. Soak shiitake (black forest) mushroom and cut into quarters. Cook in two cups of water for 15-20 minutes with a pinch of sea salt. Drink half a cup at a time.

Ume-Kuzu Drink

This drink strengthens digestion, increases vitality and can relieve general fatigue. Dissolve a heaping teaspoon of kuzu root powder into one cup of cold water. Add 1/2 of an umeboshi plum (salted plum) and a dash of shoyu (soy sauce). Bring the mixture to a boil, reduce the heat to simmering, and stir constantly until the liquid becomes a transparent gelatin. A little bit of fresh grated ginger can also be added.

Ume-Sho-Bancha

This is a macrobiotic favorite. It strengthens the blood and the circulation through the regulation of digestion. Pour one cup of bancha twig tea over the meat of 1/2 to 1 umeboshi plum and one teaspoon of tamari or soy sauce. Stir and drink hot.

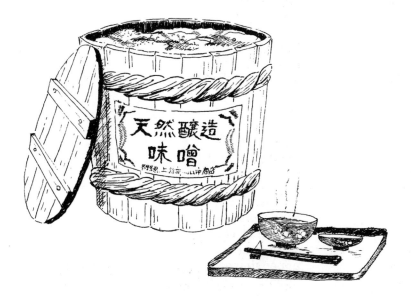

Useful Acupoints

KEY		
	HT = Heart	TH = Triple Heater
LU = Lung	SI = Small Intestine	GB = Gall Bladder
LI = Large Intestine	UB = Urinary Bladder	LV = Liver
ST = Stomach	KD = Kidney	CV = Conception Vessel
SP = Spleen	HG = Heart Governor	GV = Governing Vessel

Translated Meaning and Number of Commonly Used Acupoints

NUMBER	MEANING	LOCATION
GV 20	hundred meetings	Head and Face
Yintang	hall of the imprint	
Taiyang	highest yang	
UB 1	eyes bright	
ST 2	four white	
SI 19	listening palace	
GB 2	hearing meeting	
TH 17	screens the wind	
LI 20	welcome fragrance	
GV 26	center of man	
LU 5	foot marsh	Arms
LI 11	crooked pond	
LI 10	hand three miles	
HG 6	inner gate	
TH 5	outer gate	
LU 7	narrow defile	
LU 11	young merchant	
LI 4	joining of the valleys	
HT 7	spirit gate	
CV 13	upper stomach cavity	Abdomen
CV 12	middle stomach cavity	
CV 6	sea of energy	
CV 4	origin of the passes	
ST 25	heavenly pivot	
GB 20	wind pond	Back of Neck
GV 14	great hammer	
UB 13	lung place	Back
UB 15	heart place	

NUMBER	MEANING	LOCATION
UB 17	diaphragm place	
UB 18	liver place	
UB 19	gall bladder place	
UB 20	spleen place	
UB 21	stomach place	
UB 23	kidney place	
UB 25	large intestine place	
UB 27	small intestine place	
UB 28	urinary bladder place	
GV 4	gate of life	
GV 3	yang pass	
SP 10	sea of blood	Leg
ST 36	foot three miles	
GB 34	yang mound spring	
SP 9	yin mound spring	
SP 6	three yin crossings	
UB 54	accepting middle	
UB 57	supporting mountain	
UB 60	Kunlun mountains	Ankles
KD 3	great stream	
LV 3	supreme rushing	Feet
KD 1	bubbling spring	

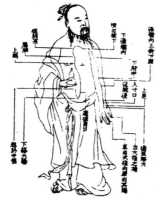

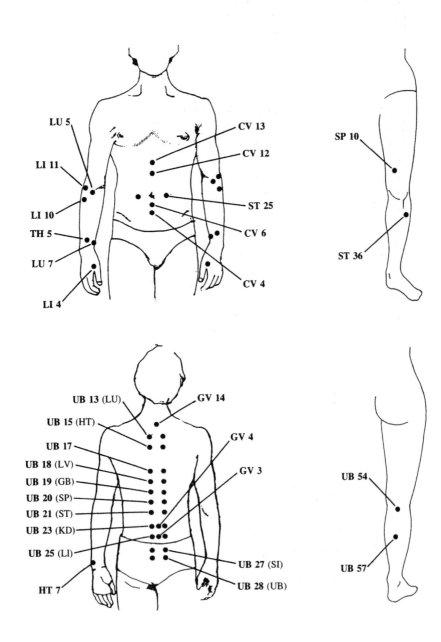

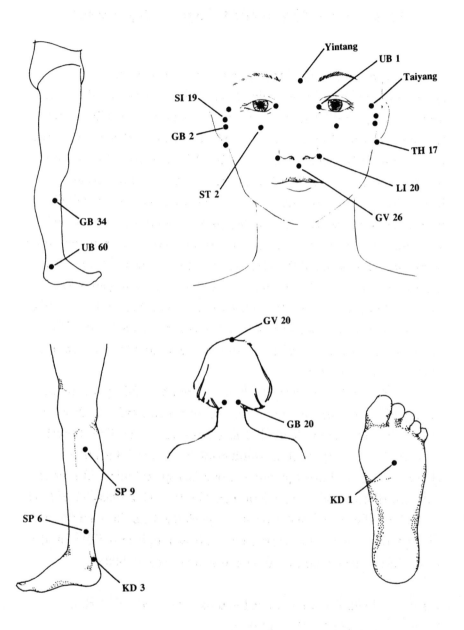

Glossary of Macrobiotic Specialty Foods

The vast majority of food items used in the macrobiotic diet (over 95%) are common everyday foods. They can be found in stores whose management has an awareness concerning quality. Varieties of whole cereal grains, such as whole wheat, barley, oats, brown rice, and so forth can be found in natural foods stores, co-ops, and in the natural foods sections of large grocery stores. Many types of beans, fresh vegetables, nuts, seeds, and fruits are also available from these same sources. For many people vegetables such as kale, kohlrabi, collard greens, dulse, turnips, and sweetmeat squash may be as foreign as some of the strange sounding names of foods that actually do originate from another country. Although you may have never tasted them before, these are common vegetables. For many of us, our choice of vegetables has been limited in the past, therefore we have unfortunately missed the array of flavors and textures that has always been available.

In macrobiotics we choose to use vegetables that grow in our immediate environment, preferably in our own gardens. Our second choice is to select those that originate from a similar climactic zone as our own—those that would grow in our area if given a chance. Some of these vegetables have foreign origins and names with which you may not be familiar. The following glossary of food items lists those commonly used as specialty foods in macrobiotics. Many have medicinal properties as well as a delicious flavor and it is for these reasons that they continue to be recommended.

Aduki is a small red bean used extensively in macrobiotics. Particularly good for the kidneys.

Agar is a sea vegetable used as a gelatin. Flavorless and very easy to use, quality agar is produced by traditional methods in clean, mountain areas, where conditions are perfect for the outdoor natural freeze-drying process.

Amazake is a very sweet rice mash which has been fermented until the rice starch has broken down into bountiful sugars. Its favorite use is as a beverage, heated with a bit of fresh ginger.

Arame, another sea vegetable, is rich in calcium and can be prepared like hijiki, though slightly sweeter in taste. It makes a wonderful tasting vegetable dish, mixed with carrots and onions. It can also be used as a tonic bath.

Bancha is a green leaf tea not normally used in macrobiotics because of its high concentration of caffeine and tannic acids. When bancha is mentioned in macrobiotic literature it is actually kukicha to which they were referring.

Daikon is a long, white radish. It is used in soups and vegetable dishes. It has the ability to dissolve unwanted accumulated matter in the body and break down fats. Particularly useful for congestion affecting the mucous membranes, such as the lung.

Hato Mugi, also known as "Job's Tears" or Pearl Barley has been recognized by traditional Chinese medicine for its ability to eliminate excessive heat from the body. Tests have shown that it rids the body of toxins, including cysts and tumors. It strengthens the spleen/pancreas systems.

Hijiki is a sea vegetable which is one of the most valuable sources of iron. It is particularly useful to promote healthy hair and skin.

Jinsei is a slightly sweet, syrupy extract, which is used to tonify the overall condition of vital organs, especially the pancreas. It is produced by slow and long cooking of juice extracted from organically grown carrots. It is believed to increase sexual vigor.

Kombu is a sea vegetable which acts as a natural flavor enhancer that is unsurpassed in making stocks for soups and sauces. Along with other sea vegetables kombu is scientifically recognized as providing assistance to the body in eliminating toxic and radioactive substances.

Kukicha (organic twig tea) is made from the two to three year-old twigs of the tea plant, which have been precisely toasted four times to remove much of the caffeine and tannic acid containing oils. The toasted twigs produce a tea which is alkaline in nature, and acts as a buffer in our digestive system.

Kuzu is a processed root vegetable used for its starch. It is particularly beneficial for the stomach and intestines and is useful in eliminating diarrhea, over acidity, and ulcers. It can be added to soups or used as a sauce.

Lotus Root is a tasty vegetable used to strengthen the lungs. It can be taken as a vegetable dish or in tea.

Mirin is cooking sake, brewed with sweet rice, well water, and a starter of sake lees. It is used in dip sauces and vegetable dishes.

Miso is a fermented soybean product which is used as a base for soups, sauces, and spreads. The best quality *miso* is made from organic beans and grains, naturally fermented in wood, aged for at least 18 months and unpasteurized. It is a good source of protein, many vitamins, iron, and other minerals.

Mochi is a versatile food made by pounding cooked sweet rice. It can be prepared by baking, frying, or in a waffle iron, it is an easy to digest grain, which can be used by everyone but with particular advantage by the sick or elderly.

Mu Tea is a mixture of either 9 or 16 ingredients used in herbal medicine. It is a delicious tea either brewed alone or with apple cider for a festive beverage.

Mugi Tea is well roasted kernels of unhulled barley. It is commonly served chilled in Japan during hot, humid summers but can also be a relaxing hot beverage during the winter.

Natto are soybeans which are inoculated, producing a fermented bean product. It is high in protein, vitamins and enzymes.

Nori is the most popular sea vegetable in Japan. It is used as an invaluable addition to soup, stew, and vegetable dishes, or as an outer wrapper of brown rice such as in sushi.

Ryusei (powdered vegetable concentrate) is prepared by gently cooking Hokkaido pumpkin, aduki beans, and kombu for up to 48 hours, and naturally drying the resultant extract. It is useful in cases of blood sugar problems.

Sake is rice wine. If you are fortunate you will find *genmai*-brown rice sake. A delicious alcoholic beverage, it can be used on festive occasions.

Seitan is a wheat gluten product that has been cooked in tamari with kombu and ginger, yielding a chewy, meat-like texture. It can be used in place of meat in all recipes such as pizza or stew.

Shiitake are mushrooms that are highly valued for their flavor and medicinal quality. They are used to lower cholesterol and to clean accumulation from the blood vessels.

Shiso is the dark red leafy vegetable found in the umeboshi package. It is from this leaf that the *ume* gets its color and flavor. Dried, it makes an excellent condiment on grains and vegetables. It is notable for its calcium content.

Shoyu (soy sauce) is brewed from whole soybeans, whole wheat, sea salt and well water and can be naturally fermented without temperature controls for more than 18 months. When purchasing *shoyu* read the label to be sure it is made without chemicals.

Soba is a delicious buckwheat pasta.

Suika-To watermelon concentrate can be used for tight kidneys. A thick, sweet extract, it is made by gently boiling down organic watermelon juice, a Japanese gourd, and cornsilk tea.

Takuan pickle are made by first washing, then, sun-drying, the daikon radish. They are packed into large wooden kegs with a special mix of rice bran and sea salt for up to one year. They are full of enzymes which aid digestion of grains.

Tamari is a wheat-free soy sauce prepared according to the same traditional methods. It is slowly matured in cedar kegs for more than one year.

Tekka is an iron-rich miso vegetable condiment made by sauteing burdock, lotus root, carrot, ginger, and hatcho miso in toasted sesame oil until somewhat dry and crumbly in texture.

Ume Concentrate is made by slowly boiling the juice of green ume fruit (similar to an apricot, however it is called a plum) for 24 hours, resulting in a very tart, alkaline extract. Dissolved in hot water or twig tea, this salt-free extract, has been used for diarrhea, constipation, dysentery, motion sickness, and other disorders of the gastro-intestinal tract.

Ume Vinegar is the liquid drawn out of the plums when they are mixed with salt to make umeboshi. Wonderful in salad dressings and sushi rice, this liquid can replace other vinegars.

Umeboshi are ume fruit which are picked green and have been pickled in salt for 12 to 18 months. Rich in enzymes, they are a valuable aid to digestion.

Wakame is a favorite sea vegetable for soup and a good introductory one, because of its mild taste.

Wasabi is the Japanese horseradish which makes traditional sushi such a festive item to eat. A little goes a long way, this hot stuff is guaranteed to spice up your life. It has been used to neutralize the toxins found in fish.

Wholewheat Fu is made from wheat gluten which has been toasted, lightly steamed, and dried. Easily reconstituted, it is a nice addition to your favorite soups and stews.

Yannoh is a grain coffee produced from aduki beans, organically grown brown rice, wheat, and chicory root.

Yansen is an extract from dandelion root which makes a strengthening tea with a beneficial effect on liver and kidneys.

Special Thanks to Blake Rankin and the Granum Company in Seattle, Washington, for assistance in providing information about macrobiotic specialty foods.

NATURAL LAWS

Seven Universal Principles

1. Everything is a different part of Infinity.
2. Everything changes.
3. All antagonisms are complementary.
4. There is nothing identical.
5. What has a front has a back.
6. The bigger the front, the bigger the back.
7. What has a beginning has an end.

Twelve Laws of Change

1. Infinity is unmistakably visible as complementary and antagonistic tendencies—Yin and Yang.
2. Yin and yang are evident continuously from the eternal movement of the universe.
3. Yin represents movement away from the center. Yang represents movement toward the center. Yin and yang together produce energy and all phenomena.
4. Yin attracts yang. Yang attracts yin.
5. Yin repels yin. Yang repels yang.
6. Yin and yang combined in varying proportions produce different visible results. The greater the difference between yin and yang forces, the greater the attraction or repulsion will be.
7. All things are transient, constantly changing their composition of yin and yang qualities; eventually yin changes into yang, yang changes into yin.
8. Nothing is solely yin nor solely yang. Everything is composed of both qualities in varying degrees.
9. There is nothing neutral. Either yin or yang is in excess in every occurrence.
10. Large yin attracts small yin. Large yang attracts small yang.
11. Extreme yin produces yang, and extreme yang produces yin.
12. All physical things are yang at the center, and yin at the surface.

INDEX

Conditions Treatable with Shiatsu

Books and Videos by the Authors

Barefoot Shiatsu
      by Shizuko Yamamoto
Barefoot Shiatsu Video
      by Shizuko Yamamoto
Releasing Tension Between the Shoulderblades (video tape)
      by Shizuko Yamamoto

Macrobiotic Shiatsu
      by Shizuko Yamamoto and Patrick McCarty

Beginner's Guide to Shiatsu
      by Patrick McCarty

These fine books and video presentations may be found at most bookstores or they may be ordered directly from:
      Turning Point Publications
      1122 "M" Street
      Eureka, CA 95501-2442
      U.S.A.
      Telephone 707-445-2290
      FAX 707-445-2391

About the Authors

Shizuko Yamamoto

Born in Japan, Ms. Yamamoto is recognized as one of the world's leading shiatsu practitioners and macrobiotic consultants. She has taught thousands of students the traditional healing art of Shiatsu. She has initiated innovative programs for the promotion of natural healing, most recently a practitioners training program. She has dedicated herself to spreading the simple message of living according to nature. To further world-wide communication in the natural healing field, she initiated the International Macrobiotic Shiatsu Society. She is the President of the Macrobiotic Center of New York in Manhattan. She has authored several books and has shared her expertise for over 30 years. She maintains an active teaching and treatment schedule in the United States and Europe.

Patrick McCarty

A native of California, Mr. McCarty is director of Ms. Yamamoto's practitioners training program. He co-directs the East-West Center for Macrobiotics, a natural health education organization in Eureka, California. His educational background includes attendance at University of California at Berkeley, Humboldt State University, and University of Málaga, Spain. He also attended the Shanghai College of Traditional Chinese Medicine in the People's Republic of China where he studied acupuncture. He edited *Barefoot Shiatsu* by Ms. Yamamoto and is the editor of "Healthways" the newsletter of the International Macrobiotic Shiatsu Society with affiliates around the world.